RESEARCH ON HUMAN SUBJECTS

Research on Human Subjects

PROBLEMS OF SOCIAL CONTROL
IN MEDICAL EXPERIMENTATION

Bernard Barber
John J. Lally
Julia Loughlin Makarushka
Daniel Sullivan

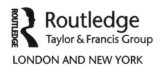

Routledge
Taylor & Francis Group

LONDON AND NEW YORK

First published 1979 by Transaction Publishers

Published 2017 by Routledge
2 Park Square, Milton Park, Abingdon, Oxon OX14 4RN
711 Third Avenue, New York, NY 10017, USA

Routledge is an imprint of the Taylor & Francis Group, an informa business

New material this edition copyright © 1979 by Taylor & Francis
Original material copyright © 1973 Russell Sage Foundation

Library of Congress Catalog Number: 77-55938

Library of Congress Cataloging in Publication Data
Main entry under title:

Research on human subjects.

Includes bibliographical references and index.
1. Human experimentation in medicine—Moral and religious aspects. 2. Human experimentation in medicine—Social aspects. 3. Social control. I. Barber, Bernard.
R853.H8R47 1978   174'.2   78-55938
ISBN 0-87855-649-4

ISBN 13: 978-0-87855-649-6 (pbk)

CONTENTS

PREFACE TO THE PAPERBACK EDITION

With the perspective of five years since the original publication of this book in 1973, we would like to do two things in this preface to the paperback edition that should be of interest to the reader. First, we would like to assess, at least in a limited way, how well our findings have held up in view of consequent work. In particular, we now have in hand the Cooke-Tannenbaum-Gray report[1] to the National Commission for the Protection of Human Subjects (hereafter just the National Commission) which is based on comprehensive interview surveys of members of Institutional Review Boards (IRB's), investigators involved in research with human subjects, and former research subjects and proxies. Each of us had a small influence on the design of that study, and we tried to make sure that analyses of those data could serve as checks on some of the conclusions reported in our book.[2] There are only a few other relevant empirical studies to which ours can be compared, and we will try to mention them where appropriate.

Second, for those who have an interest in how a book such as ours does and does not find its way effectively into the policy-making process, we review here the extent of our success in making our ideas visible, in getting some of them accepted, and in getting an even smaller number enacted. Those duties have been taken up primarily by the senior author (B.B.), but all of us have participated to various degrees. There is much policy yet to be made, and perhaps the wider circulation which this paperback edition will provide our book will enhance the dialogue still in progress.

ASSESSMENT

Is There a Problem?

In chapter 3 of our book, we presented analyses of the expressed ethical standards with respect to the use of human subjects held by respondents to two surveys, a national survey of biomedical research institutions and an intensive two-institution study, and analyses of the risks and benefits of the 424 research projects involving human subjects being conducted at the time by the researchers we interviewed in the two-institution study. In the case of expressed ethical standards we found that, in evaluating hypothetical research protocols which we had designed so that they would involve the ethical dilemmas at issue here, a significant minority of respondents to each question approved of studies that were highly questionable to the majority. For example, one hypothetical question, involving thymectomies in children undergoing open heart surgery, was essentially a version of the hotly debated study by Zollinger et al. done at Children's Hospital Medical Center in 1964.[3] Twenty-one percent of the respondents in our national survey would have approved of that study if they were a review committee of one if there were a 50 percent chance or less that an important scientific discovery would result. Data of that kind suggested that there was no full consensus in the biomedical research community on the ethical standards that should guide human experimentation, and also led us to conclude that a significant minority of researchers held quite "permissive" standards.

The National Commission survey asked a large sample of investigators (N = 1660) whose research involved human subjects whether eleven research practices were acceptable.[4] Their study included behavioral scientists and "other" investigators, but the responses of the biomedical scientists (N = 1040) were broken out separately. While none of the research practices mentioned was similar in all ways to any of our hypothetical research proposals, it is fair to conclude, we feel, that the overall pattern is quite similar. Seven years after our data were collected, there is still no detailed consensus among biomedical researchers on appropriate ethical standards, except perhaps in the area of keeping information about subjects confidential. This value, of course, is closely tied to traditional standards among physicians involving confidentiality with respect to patient records. A significant fraction of this nationally representative sample of investigators seems quite permissive in their standards.

With respect to the risks and benefits of research, there are some interesting differences between the results from our two-institution study and the research sponsored by the National Commission. Our two institutions, an elite medical-school/teaching-hospital complex and an urban community and teaching hospital, were certainly not representative of all sites in which biomedical research on humans is done, but they were quite typical of centers in which a large volume of such human experimentation is done. We obtained data on all research projects involving humans in which our interview respondents (72 percent of all researchers involved in human experimentation in the two institutions) were engaged, a total of 424 in all. Forty-four percent of the projects were reported to have no risk of physical harm whatsoever and only 17 percent were said to involve "little or no" therapeutic benefit to the subjects.

The National Commission researchers obtained data on a representative sample of projects involving human subjects at 61 institutions. There were 1,272 biomedical projects in the sample, and 31 percent[5] of them were reported by the investigators to be "non-beneficial" while 32 percent[6] were classified as having no risk of even minor medical complications. If anything, then, our data understate the amount of risk involved in biomedical human experimentation and overstate the probability of benefit.

Our data on the issue of informed consent to participation as a research subject are not extensive. They are limited largely to responses by the researchers we surveyed in our studies to the hypothetical research proposals, mentioned earlier, in which informed consent was an issue. We found diversity of opinion among researchers about the conditions under which consent was required and, if required, how it should be obtained, but the commission study is much more comprehensive in this area. In addition to asking many questions of investigators and IRB members about what they felt ought to happen in this area, the commission researchers analyzed the written consent forms actually used in over 1,600 studies to see how they reflected what was to be done in the research. Also, 809 subjects and 153 proxies were interviewed. The commission researchers caution that this sample of subjects and proxies is not representative "of the larger population of research participants and/or their proxies," but the results are suggestive nonetheless.

Their results here are too numerous to detail, but a few can be mentioned to indicate the general nature of the findings. "Approximately 10 percent of the respondents said that they did not understand before their participation actually began that they were to be involved in research."[7] "Eighty-three percent of the subjects and proxies reported that someone connected with the study talked with them and told them what was going to be done."[8] Only 8 percent of the subjects interviewed said that deciding to be a subject was a "somewhat" or "very difficult" decision.[9] No analyses are reported whose goal is to explain variance in the experiences reported by subjects, however, and so Gray's earlier cast study[10] remains the definitive published analysis of the structural pressures which lead to the incompleteness or nonexistence of informed consent.

We also reported in chapter 3 that studies with the least favorable risks-benefits ratios were more likely to involve ward and clinic patients than private patients. Since ward and clinic patients are differentially poor, less educated, and members of minority groups, and since Gray's studies[11] revealed that such groups much less frequently are able to (or are helped to) give a free and informed consent, these findings were disturbing to us. The National Commission study "did not find that children, women, minority or low income persons were more likely than others to participate in projects that were above average in risk. Nor were they less likely than others to participate in projects that were intended to benefit the subject."[12] But the commission data are very underanalyzed at this point, and it is much too soon to conclude that we were mistaken in what we feel is a finding that is generally true of biomedical research. The commission researchers did not construct a "risks-benefits ratio" from data such as that in their Table

XV.21,[13] for example, but relied instead on statements made by the researchers who were interviewed about whether the risks exceeded the benefits in their research (see their Table XV.23).[14] We would like to see much more analysis of this important issue by the commission researchers. We concluded in our chapter 3 that there is a problem with the way in which research on human subjects is conducted, and no new data have emerged to indicate that we were mistaken.

Effects of Competition in Scientific Community and Local and Scientific Reward Systems

Our analyses in chapters 4 and 5 of the effects of scientific competition and of local-institutional and scientific reward systems on the probability that an investigator would undertake a study with a less favorable risks-benefits ratio for subjects have not been replicated. We found that researchers who did not do well in the scientific or in the local-institutional competition for rewards were more likely than others to be involved in studies with less favorable risks-benefits ratios for subjects. These analyses, though tentative in part, remain unchallenged and, so far as we know, the relationship between the structure and functioning of the biomedical research community and the way human subjects are used in research is not receiving any attention in policy. The research community is itself pathogenic, at least to a degree, and perhaps we will never adequately regulate the use of humans in research until we better understand the pathology. The National Commission research would, with suitable new data collection, be made into a much better study of these questions than our study, and we strongly urge that appropriate steps be taken.

Socialization

A third area of concern in our research was the extent and consequences of any socialization into the ethical standards involved in human experimentation that was experienced by the investigators interviewed in our two-institution study (chapters 6 and 7). We wanted to assess the extent to which the typical career of a biomedical researcher involves formal and informal occasions to learn an appropriate set of ethical standards for human experimentation, and then we wanted to see if researchers who had had such opportunities for "moral learning" behaved any differently in their current research. We found that recent medical school graduates were more likely to report ethically socializing experiences in medical school, a trend that is substantiated by the Veatch-Sollitto survey.[15] We also found that investigators who reported having had such experiences in medical school or at other junctures in their career were only somewhat less likely than others to have "permissive" ethical standards, though cause and effect is unclear, and also were only slightly less likely to be involved in studies with less favorable risks-benefits ratios. The latter finding, however, was an interaction effect, which is to say that having had early socialization experiences only affected the behavior of our researchers when, in addition, they fell into a particular category of a third variable. The effects of ethical socialization, or prior moral learning during medical training, on behavior were therefore quite small.

Such an outcome was undoubtedly due, in part, to the unplanned and unintegrated nature of most of that ethical socialization, combined with the relatively large emphasis in medical education on the value of science and on the professional autonomy of the individual physician and scientist. But also, it is illuminated by learning theory.[16] Norms learned at one stage in a person's life, if not subsequently and periodically reinforced, will eventually decline in importance as determinants of behavior. Evidence from our study and others indicates that powerful reinforcements of ethical learning have been rare in the situations in which biomedical research on human subjects is practiced. The settings of biomedical research on humans are highly structured, and situational pressures on behavior are very strong. But the pressures seem to be much more in the direction of the value of science than they are in support of the ethical and humane treatment of human subjects. Those ethical values researchers do have remain unreinforced while competing values (the value of science and of professional autonomy) are emphasized.

However, direct intervention in or close social regulation of medical research settings in order to safeguard research subjects would itself violate deeply held values of the medical profession and perhaps have ramifying and unforeseen negative consequences for medical science. Any realistic system to protect subjects must depend in some part on the ethical predispositions of research physicians, not only for the ethical conduct of their own research, but also for effective formal or informal peer control of each other.

Thus we still maintain, as we did in our chapter 11, that *both* internalized standards and external controls, such as IRB's, are needed, and that improvement and invention are required in respect to both. However, it is clearer now that such improvements, if they are not to be governmentally imposed, but yet are to be effective, require that significant changes be instituted by the medical profession itself in the social structure, culture, reward system, and processes of medical educational and work settings— changes which seem largely not to have been made during the five years since our book first appeared.[17]

Again, however, our analyses in this area have not been replicated in any way. Data collected as part of the National Commission study may shed further light on these questions, but analyses performed so far have not addressed this area of our work.

Institutional Review Boards and Peer Review

Our book reports the results of the first national survey of the structure and functioning of the Institutional Review Boards (IRB's), required by the Public Health Service in 1966. These local-institutional committees, which had to be established in every institution in which research on human subjects was being done with PHS money, were to look to three problems in every piece of research using human subjects that was supported by PHS funds: (1) the rights and welfare of the subject; (2) the appropriateness of the methods of getting consent; and (3) the risks and potential benefits of the investigation. Our data, accurate for the year 1969, have now been comprehensively updated to 1976 by the National Commission study. Their data on the structure and functioning of IRB's for 1976 are much more detailed and comprehensive than ours for 1969, and in addition they conducted interviews with over 800 members of review boards in 61 institutions. Further, they examined research protocols before and after review by the IRB's to see what impact the committees had had.

The new results of the commission study are far too numerous to mention here. Where there is direct overlap between our analyses and theirs, the results are very similar. For example, in both studies, the more active the IRB, the less well accepted it was by investigators in the institution. The commission study clearly must be seen as the best source for current information about IRB's, their composition, functioning, and impact. Our study, however, gives a better view of the early stages of this new social innovation, particularly of the different ways this new regulation was handled by different types of institutions. Specifically, our analysis of the lack of leadership in this area by medical schools, in chapter 10, remains an important insight into the resistant role medical schools played at the onset of increased governmental regulation.

In summary, where our analyses have been replicated they have held up well. In some areas (informed consent, structure and functioning of IRB's, and overall generality) our work has been considerably extended. But in other areas, mainly where we have endeavored to explain variations in the attitudes or behavior of biomedical researchers, there have been few new analyses and few new data. It remains a puzzle to us that so few researchers have joined in our efforts to understand how the research system which includes human experimentation actually works. Hundreds of people have written in recent years about what ought to be the standards in this area, but only a handful have tried to understand better the empirical situation to which all proposed new standards would apply. We have long felt that attempts at policy change or policy development in the absence of such an understanding were vacuous, and while the National Commission did undertake extensive empirical research of the necessary kind, it remains underanalyzed and, as a result, less useful for policy.

SOCIAL POLICY AND SOCIAL CHANGE

We turn now to what we have learned from the fate of the results of our book in the social and political arena. We think we have acquired some useful new knowledge, or at least some old knowledge in a new way, about the limited effects of knowledge on the making of social policy and about the complex processes of social change. Early on in our research, realizing that our findings might have implications for social policy, we resolved to make some explicit recommendations for improved policy on the matter of research on human subjects. On the basis of our findings, therefore, especially those about sources of strain and defects in the existing system, we wrote a last chapter (11) entitled "The Social Responsibilities of a Powerful Profession: Some Suggestions for Policy Change and Reform." In that chapter, we emphasized the adverse consequences of the dilemma of science and humane therapy, and we suggested specific changes in the structures and procedures of medical school education, of postgraduate medical training and research, and particularly of the local institutional peer review boards.

Our fond hope was that the "powerful profession" we addressed would be both attentive to our recommendations, and active and constructive in initiating the proposed changes. We should have known better. Except for scattered exceptions, medical researchers paid little attention to our book and continued in their established ways of considerable indifference and a small amount of hostility to those who said that all was not well with their practices in the use of human subjects. Even the few critical "insiders" who agreed with us that something was wrong did not see that it was the *system* of medical education and peer consultation that was responsible for the existing defects. For example, even someone like the late Professor Henry Beecher of the Harvard Medical School, whose 1966 article in the *Journal of the American Medical Association* describing some twenty-five articles in the professional medical and research journals that showed evidence of unethical use of human subjects stunned his colleagues into some awareness of the problem, thought in individualistic, psychologistic terms.[18] He thought he was dealing with just a few "bad guys," a small number of defective individuals within the medical research community. But our whole point was that it was a "bad system" that was turning a lot of "good guys" into "bad guys."[19]

We have said we should have known better than to expect much self-reform from our "powerful profession." On sociological grounds, we should have expected what in fact occurred, that they would resist the proposed changes, that they would be conservative in the literal sense, that is, unwilling to change the status quo. All social groups tend to be conservative when they feel that their central values and interests are being challenged or are in danger of being subverted. For the medical research community, the changes that we and others proposed seemed like illegitimate challenges to their values and interests with regard to autonomy and hard-earned expertise. Just as powerful businessmen in the past resisted, and still do, the "encroachments" of government on their autonomy and self-defined expertise, so the medical research community today feels itself beleaguered by an excessively intrusive general public and the government as well. Even small requests for change, for more effective self-regulation, are viewed by the "powerful profession" as fundamental threats.

Slowly we came to the conclusion that only further government action would push the medical research community toward the necessary reforms. By coincidence, just about this time, there was much concern in government circles and among the public about the ethics of the use of human subjects as a result of much newspaper publicity about the "Tuskegee scandal." Crusading journalists had reported that a group of poor black men in Tuskegee, Alabama had been used as subjects in a syphilis experiment without their informed consent and without their being given the best presently available treatment. The "Tuskegee scandal" aroused the attention and the action of Senator Edward Kennedy, the chairman of the Senate Health and Science Subcommittee. We were asked, on the basis of the findings reported in our book, to testify before the subcommittee on a bill he had introduced to set up a National Commission for the Protection of the Human Subjects of Biomedical and Behavioral Research. Our views on the necessity for government initiatives were expressed in the following way:

> Is Government regulation necessary? Why not leave control of these matters to the researchers themselves? I want to answer this question if only because I know it will be asked by some of the researchers who will appear before you and who will speak in favor of professional autonomy. That is only to be expected. All powerful professional groups resist objective scrutiny and control by outsiders and pledge that their own wisdom, initiative, and compassion are sufficient to protect the interests and values of their clients. But my answer is different. I think so because it is a fact, carefully demonstrated by our research findings, that the research professions have not taken the initiatives necessary for protecting their human subjects. They have tended only to respond, and then reluctantly, to Government mandate enforced by the power of the purse. They have been laggard in improving the ethical education of their students, undistinguished in using peer review to

control questionable research, and relatively more interested in the demands of scientific achievement than in the obligations of humane treatment of subjects.[20]

Since the bill to establish the National Commission did eventually become law and the commission was set up and has been functioning for three years, we ask what part our knowledge and that of others played in this outcome. Moral outrage over the "Tuskegee scandal" and political action by the Congress were of course the major determinants of this result, but knowledge did play some part. First, the bill itself was based on a draft that had been prepared for other reasons by two experts in the field of research on human subjects, Professor Jay Katz, a psychiatrist on the Yale Law School faculty, and his then-associate, Professor Alexander Capron, now of the University of Pennsylvania Law School. Second, our research findings, given in detail to the subcommittee, played a part in showing that the defects exposed at Tuskegee were system-wide in medical research and that reform was not likely to be forthcoming from researchers themselves.

Although we had come to feel that government action was necessary and were pleased that the National Commission had been established, we knew that such action was not enough by itself to bring about the reforms we thought essential. Government action by itself is seldom sufficient for effective social change. Change has to result from action in several social and normative modes, each reenforcing the others toward some common desired outcome. On the moral and normative side, for example, we were glad to see the emergence of what has come to be called the "bioethics movement."[21] This is a movement made up of change agents from the fields of ethics, philosophy, the law, and the humanities, all concerned with improving the moral use and treatment of people by medical practitioners and researchers. The "bioethicists" have held conferences, written books and papers, given lectures, held seminars, provided training facilities for all those newly interested in medical ethics, and even established specialized action and study institutes for this field. Our own efforts to bring about the proposed social changes have also been multisided. We have consulted with foundations making research grants, lectured to medical and lay audiences, spoken on television, advised newspaper reporters, helped young researchers in the field, attended conferences, coached lawyers bringing suits on behalf of prisoner subjects, met with social workers concerned for their medical clients, served on advisory boards of research and action organizations, helped to construct new professional codes of ethics, written further articles and book reviews, arranged professional discussions, and visited with researchers interested in these problems in such places as England, Sweden, India, the Philippines, Colombia, and Brazil. The processes of social change, we have learned from all this, are slow, not easy to come by,

xvi • RESEARCH ON HUMAN SUBJECTS

from some effective combination of moral, organizational, legal, governmental, and personal changes.

A few words in conclusion. The treatment of human subjects in biomedical research has been noticeably improved during the last fifteen years, perhaps chiefly as a result of government action but helped along by the bioethics movement and by the knowledge produced by social research like ours. Yet much remains to be done. There is room for improvement in the functioning of the local institutional peer review boards and in the effectiveness of medical education. Social change is on its way, but not yet completed.

BERNARD BARBER
JOHN J. LALLY
JULIA LOUGHLIN MAKARUSHKA
DANIEL SULLIVAN

February 1978

NOTES

1. Robert A. Cooke, Arnold S. Tannenbaum, and Bradford Gray, *A Survey of Institutional Review Boards and Research Involving Human Subjects* (Ann Arbor: Survey Research Center, University of Michigan, 1977).

2. The commission research is, of course, much more than just a check on our findings. It breaks much new ground in terms of content, but especially in terms of scope, comprehensiveness, and representativeness. Data on the use of human subjects in *behavioral* research have been collected for the first time, for example.

3. See Robert M. Zollinger, Jr., et al., "Effect of Thymectomy on Skin-Homograft Survival in Children," *New England Journal of Medicine* 270 (1964): 707–09 for details of the study. See Jay Katz, *Experimentation With Human Beings* (New York: Russell Sage, 1972), pp. 960–62 for the nature of the debate.

4. See Table XVII.3, Cooke et al., p. 239. For example, is "high risk research of considerable importance in which there is no direct benefit to subjects but they are fully informed and capable of given consent" acceptable?

5. See Table XV.1, ibid., p. 209.

6. See Table XV.16, ibid., p. 224.

7. Ibid., p. 70.

8. Ibid., p. 71.

9. Ibid., p. 71.

10. Bradford H. Gray, *Human Subjects in Medical Experimentation* (New York: Wiley, Interscience, 1975).

11. Ibid., pp. 56–84.

12. Cooke et al., p. *ix*.

13. Ibid., p. 230.

14. Ibid., p. 233.

15. Robert M. Veatch and Sharmon Sollitto, "Medical Ethics Teaching: A Report of a National Medical School Survey," *Journal of the American Medical Association* 235 (1976): 1030–33.

16. See, for example, John Finley Scott, *The Internalization of Norms* (Englewood Cliffs, N.J.: Prentice-Hall, 1971), ch. 3.

17. Regarding medical education, see John J. Lally, "The Making of the Compassionate Physician-Investigator," *Medical Ethics and Social Change*, ed. Bernard Barber, and *Annals of the American Academy of Political and Social Science* 437, (1978); see also Rue Bucher and Joan G. Stelling, *Becoming Professional* (Beverly Hills, Calif.: Sage, 1977), esp. pp. 279–85 and the Preface by Eliot Freidson.

18. Henry K. Beecher, "Consent in Clinical Experimentation: Myth and Reality," *Journal of the American Medical Association* 194 (1966): 34–35.

19. For the details of our argument, see Bernard Barber, "Compassion in Medicine: Toward New Definitions and New Institutions," *New England Journal of Medicine* 295 (1976): 939–43; and John J. Lally and Bernard Barber. "The Compassionate Physician: Frequency and Social Determinants of Physician-Investigator Concern for Human Subjects," *Social Forces* 53 (1974): 289–96.

20. Bernard Barber, "Prepared Statement," Senate Subcommittee on Health and Science, Hearings on Protection of Human Subjects Act, June 28, 1973.

21. On this see Renee C. Fox, "Advanced Medical Technology—Social and Ethical Implications," *Annual Review of Sociology* (1976): 231–68.

PREFACE

This book is intended for at least two types of reader: those who are primarily interested in the ethical problems connected with the use of human subjects in biomedical experimentation and our fellow professional sociologists. Readers of the first type will look immediately to our substantive findings and to our policy recommendations, but we hope they also will pay attention to our sociological analysis and our empirical research methods. We are convinced that our findings and policy recommendations are possible only because of our sociological analysis and methods. We are further convinced that in this area of ethical problems of human experimentation, as in all other social problems areas, we must transcend even the best of available lay "wisdom" by the use of technical and tested theory and research. We hope that some of these readers will become similarly convinced and will help to sponsor and support further research.

Our second type of reader will be fellow professional sociologists. Since sociologists are becoming increasingly specialized and therefore increasingly insular in their research and interests, it is necessary to make explicit the different specialized sociological interests we had to bring together in writing this book. We have, of course, had to marry theory and research with the closest bonds. The result, as might be expected, has been a considerable increase in mutual productiveness. At a few points at least, we feel our research has made it possible for us to clarify matters of sociological theory. For example, we hope this is the case in our discussion of the relation between social structure and culture, in our discussion of the theory of social deviance, and in our discussion of the theory of professional socialization. Of course, we had to use a great deal of the analyses and findings of those two flourishing sociological specialties, the sociology of science and the sociology of medicine. And, finally, we know that specialists in the sociology of the professions will find materials and analyses of interest here.

It is a pleasure to acknowledge some of the debts we have acquired in this extensive and complex undertaking and to give thanks for help received from several people. Orville G. Brim, Jr., then president of Russell Sage Foundation, and Howard E. Freeman, a member of the staff of Russell Sage Foundation, have been helpful throughout the several years of our work. Dr. Donald T. Chalkley and his colleagues of the Division of Research Grants of the National Institutes of Health were encouraging of our project from its beginning and provided the necessary lists of biomedical research organizations. On the medical side, giving counsel on essential technical matters in that area, Dr. Louis Lasagna, Dr. John F. Bertles, and Dr. George G. Reader have been invaluable. Our Columbia sociology colleagues, Jonathan Cole and Charles Kadushin, gave us essential methodological guidance. Elaine Samuel was a key member of our interviewing staff in our Intensive Two-Institution Study. So too was Leslie Barber, who "dropped in" to work with us for a year and did a dozen different tasks with unfailing grace and efficiency. Lily Soohoo spent several academic terms and summers as an indispensable administrative and research assistant. Gail Freedman helped us out as a research assistant toward the end of our work. We are, of course, enormously grateful to the hundreds of busy medical researchers who took the time to answer our questionnaire or be interviewed in person. Finally, to our spouses—Elinor, Mary, Chrys, and Ann—we give thanks for the help which directly and indirectly contributed to our work.

BERNARD BARBER
JOHN J. LALLY
New York   JULIA LOUGHLIN MAKARUSHKA
November 1972   DANIEL SULLIVAN

1

INTRODUCTION

All during this century, but with especial frequency during the last thirty years, a large number of discoveries have been made in biomedical science. The area of therapeutic drug discovery and use may perhaps serve as an example of what is happening in many other areas of biomedicine. Three of what are now the eight major classes of prescribed therapeutic drugs were unknown thirty years ago. These three are the antibiotics, the antihistamines, and the psychoactive drugs. Two other major classes of drugs, the sulfas and vitamins, were introduced between World Wars I and II. Somewhat earlier in the century, barbiturates and hormones were discovered. In sum, of the eight major classes of prescribed therapeutic drugs, only narcotic drugs were known to antiquity, and today's representatives of even this class, with the exception of morphine and codeine, are recently developed drugs.[1]

Accompanying this rapid progress in biomedicine, indeed a prerequisite for it, has been a very large and very rapid increase in the amount of use of human subjects in biomedical research. Although research starts in the laboratory and then proceeds to animal testing, eventually all new procedures, new techniques, new drugs have to be tested for efficacy in man. As Dr. Henry Beecher, a pioneer among those concerned for the ethics of research, has put it, man is "the final test site." Or, in other words, "man is the animal of necessity" in this situation.

Of course, all this successful biomedical research on human subjects has enormously benefited the health and welfare of those who enjoy modern medical care anywhere in the world. However, as with probably all purposive social action, there have also been some unintended and undesired side-effects, in both the medical and the moral realms.[2] Chief among the undesired moral side-effects has been the apparent failure to achieve the highest, and in

---

[1] Further on the subject of drug discovery and use, and on the sociology of drugs in general, see Bernard Barber, *Drugs and Society* (New York: Russell Sage Foundation, 1967).

[2] For a discussion and further references on these effects in the medical realm, see *Ibid.*, multiple references in Index under "adverse effects."

many cases even adequate, standards of professional moral concern and behavior with the human subjects used in this necessary biomedical experimentation. At the center of our interest in this book are the social sources of
satisfactory and unsatisfactory standards of concern and practice with human subjects.

Although there has been a rather long history of attention to the problem of the possible or actual abuse of the subjects of medical innovation and
medical experimentation, this attention has increased a great deal during the
last ten years or so.[3] First, increased attention and concern were expressed
from within the biomedical research community itself.[4] A little later, a number of biomedical researchers, joined by professors of law, moral philosophy, and social science, organized symposia to compose a rounded view of
the problem.[5] The recent increase of concern in the biomedical research
community can be seen perhaps most clearly in the dramatic rise of medical
journal articles devoted to facets of this problem. If we look at *Index Medicus*, we find an increase in both the absolute number and the proportion of
articles in this area. Table 1.1 documents the results of our count of all those
articles listed under the headings "Ethics, medical" and "Human Experimen-

---

[3] For an historical anthology of expressions of this concern, see Irving Ladimer and
Roger W. Newman, eds., *Clinical Investigation in Medicine* (Boston: Boston University
Law-Medicine Research Institute, 1963). A turning point in the development of concern
was the Nuremberg trials of Nazi doctors who abused their human subjects. The Nuremberg Code and many subsequent codes were the outcome of these trials. A large collection of these codes appear in Henry K. Beecher, *Research and the Individual: Human
Studies* (Boston: Little, Brown, 1970).

[4] Dr. Henry K. Beecher has been writing from within and to the biomedical research community since at least 1953. See his "Clinical Impression and Clinical Investigation," *Journal of the American Medical Association*, 151 (1953): 44-45. See also his *Experimentation in Man* (Springfield, Ill.: Charles C. Thomas, 1959) and *Research and the
Individual: Human Studies* (Boston: Little, Brown, 1970). The British equivalent of
Beecher may be found in M. H. Pappworth, *Human Guinea Pigs* (London: Routledge
and Kegan Paul, 1967; Boston: Beacon Press, 1967). For a sampling of responses to
Beecher's work by members of the biomedical research community, see *New England
Journal of Medicine*, 275 (1966): 790-791. These followed the publication of an article
by Beecher in that journal. For alleged unethical use of human subjects in Italy, see
Medical Tribune, Dec. 22, 1971 and Jan. 26, 1972.

[5] See the results of these symposia in *Daedalus*, 98, No. 2 (1969), and *Annals of the
New York Academy of Sciences*, 169 (Jan. 21, 1970). See also G. E. W. Wolstenholme
and Maeve O'Connor, eds., *Ethics in Medical Progress* (Boston: Little, Brown, 1966). For
earlier expressions of our own interest in this area, see Bernard Barber, "Experimenting
With Humans," *The Public Interest*, no. 6 (Winter, 1968): 91-102; Bernard Barber, "New
Ethical Procedures in the Professions," *Journal of the American Pharmaceutical Associa-
tion*, NS8 (March, 1968): 137-140; and Bernard Barber, "Some 'New Men of Power':
The Case of Biomedical Research Scientists," in *Annals of the New York Academy of
Sciences*, 169 (Jan. 21, 1970): 519-522.

Table 1.1. Number and Proportion of Articles on Human Experimentation by Year and Type of Journal

Year	Number of Articles		Number Indexed/ 100,000 Articles Indexed	
	English Lang.	Foreign Lang.	English Lang.	Foreign Lang.
1950	0	0	0.0	0.0
1960	2	0	1.6	0.0
1965	6	1	3.5	0.6
1966	20	3	12.1	1.8
1967	30	1	18.2	0.6
1968	41	4	19.8	1.9
1969	21	11	9.4	4.9

tation" whose titles indicate that they are indeed on the subject of the ethics of biomedical research on human subjects. It will be observed that the figures begin to get large in 1966, when the classificatory heading "Human Experimentation" first appeared in *Index Medicus* and when the U.S. Public Health Service first issued its requirements and guidelines to grantee institutions for safeguarding the rights and welfare of human subjects. The figures are given for both foreign-language and English-language journals and they indicate considerably greater concern in the English-language world.

It should be noted that all articles on the subject of the ethical problems of tissue transplantation were excluded from Table 1.1. Transplantation in its early phases involves the use of experimental human subjects, of course, but it includes other ethical problems as well, for example, the ethical problem of when "life" should be ended. That is why it is indexed separately. Although tissue transplantation has been a highly publicized issue in the last few years, especially since the first heart transplants, the articles on transplantation specifically are fewer than half as many as those on experimentation more generically. In 1950 and 1960 there were no articles indexed on tissue transplantation. Table 1.2 shows the figures for 1965 to 1969.

Second, increased attention and concern have been expressed in new governmental regulations, most powerfully in those of the National Institutes of Health and the Food and Drug Administration.[6] Because they have mandated peer review for all biomedical research that they have supported since 1966, which includes a considerable part of all the biomedical research done in the United States as a whole and in nearly every individual biomedical re-

---

[6] For a detailed account of the development of these regulations, see William J. Curran, "The Approach of Two Federal Agencies," *Daedalus*, 98, no. 2 (1969): 542–594.

Table 1.2. Number of Articles Indexed on Tissue Transplantation

Year	Number of Articles in English Language Journals
1965	3
1966	4
1967	3
1968	13
1969	17

search organization, the National Institutes of Health have played an especially important role in the regulation of the use of human subjects.[7] The scope of governmental regulation in the biomedical and other human experimental areas has been steadily increasing. In 1971, the Food and Drug Administration, which up to that point had required only written voluntary consent from subjects, added the requirement of peer review for all clinical research. And in 1971 also, the Department of Health, Education, and Welfare moved its control over the use of human subjects to a higher level than that of its subdepartment, the National Institutes of Health. The Department's Office of Grant Administration Policy has been given authority for "establishing uniform policies for the protection of human subjects involved in research, demonstration, and other activities supported by the Department's grants and contracts."[8] Although determination of the applicability of the policy is left to the professional judgment of the operating agencies involved, the policy is now supposed to cover *all* psychological, sociological, and educational research using human subjects and "certainly includes all medical research." The Department's new uniform policies have been stated in the Office of Grants Administration Manual, Chapter 1–40, and this statement on "Protection of Human Subjects," now supersedes the 1969 N.I.H. regulation, "Protection of the Individual as a Research Subject."

---

[7] For one version of its regulations in this area, see U.S. Department of Health, Education, and Welfare—Public Health Service, *Protection of the Individual as a Research Subject* (Washington, D.C.: U.S. Government Printing Office, 1969).

[8] *DRG Newsletter*, May, 1971 (published by the National Institutes of Health). The final policy can be found in *The Institutional Guide to DHEW Policy on Protection of Human Subjects*, Washington, D.C. (U.S. Government Printing Office), Dec. 1, 1971. Except for Austria, the United States is the only country in the world with specific legislation in this area. According to a letter from Dr. J. De Moerlooze of the Health Legislation Unit of the World Health Organization (personal communication), "The situation in the United States where . . . specific regulations have been issued . . . virtually constitutes an exception to the general pattern. In fact, legal provisions dealing with experimentation are, as a rule, non-existent in the world today."

Third and finally, increased attention and concern have been widely and continually displayed in the mass media. This concern has been especially focused on three causes célèbres during the last ten years: the thalidomide disaster in Germany; the Southam and Mandel case in New York State in which live cancer cells were injected into geriatric patients without their informed consent; and the bitter controversy between Drs. DeBakey and Cooley of Baylor University and Houston over their own priority rights and the rights of patients in their artificial heart and heart transplant programs.[9]

Unfortunately, all this literature of concern, both past and present, has some important defects. Though often wise, it contains a paucity of hard and detailed facts based on representative samples of experience. Also, it lacks the understanding of some of the sources of possible ethical shortcomings in this area which can be provided by sociological analysis. Finally, because of its inadequate factual basis and its unsatisfactory analysis, the policy recommendations made in this literature have often been limited or defective. The purpose of the studies and the work carried out over a period of several years by our Research Group on Human Experimentation has been to make improvements in all these respects: to provide better facts, better analysis, and better policy recommendations.

The extensive details of our empirical findings, our sociological analysis, and our policy recommendations are presented in this book. Here, as a guide to the reader, we offer a prospect of what our book contains, a brief and synoptic outline presented to help keep the macroscopic picture in view when we come to focus on the microscopic detail that is of its essence.

Since our work represents the first attempt ever to obtain systematic empirical estimates on both expressed ethical standards and actual behavioral practices with regard to the use of human subjects in biomedical experimentation, we start with a detailed account of the design and methodology of the two studies in which we collected our data.[10] The careful reader of a sci-

---

[9] For information on the thalidomide birth defects, see United States Senate, Report of the Committee on Government Operations, *Interagency Drug Coordination* (Washington, D.C.: U.S. Government Printing Office, 1965). The Southam-Mandel case is documented in *Hyman v. Jewish Chronic Disease Hospital*, 251 N.Y.S. 2nd 818 (1964). Extensive excerpts from these proceedings are reprinted in Jay Katz, *Experimentation with Human Beings* (New York: Russell Sage Foundation, 1972). A publication documenting the facts in the DeBakey-Cooley controversy is promised from the American Heart Institute. For a journalistic account, see Thomas Thompson, *Hearts: Of Surgeons and Transplants, Miracles and Disasters along the Cardiac Frontier* (New York: McCall, 1971).

[10] An attempt to obtain some systematic empirical evidence on expressed standards, but not behavior, in this field can be found in Earl R. Babbie, *Science and Morality in Medicine* (Berkeley, Calif.: University of California Press, 1969), especially pp. 64–72.

entific monograph, we recognize, always looks first to see how the data were collected and measured. In this case, for example, the careful reader will want to inspect the representativeness of our samples and the validity of the instruments with which we collected data on the two key issues in this area: the issue of *informed voluntary consent* and the issue of the *proper balance between risk and benefit* in experiments done with human subjects.[11] The first of our two studies, our National Survey, obtained responses to a mailed questionnaire survey from a set of 293 biomedical research institutions which our analysis shows to constitute a nationally representative sample along several important dimensions of all American institutions of this kind.[12] The second study, our Intensive Two-Institution Study, obtained responses to lengthy personal interviews, using a different instrument from the first study, from the active researchers in two biomedical research institutions chosen by cluster analysis to be representative of a very large number of the institutions in our national sample.[13] In one of these two institutions, University Hospital and Research Center, we obtained 331 interviews or questionnaires; at the other, Community and Teaching Hospital, 56. It is likely that, because of our high response rate (72%) and because of the method of selecting these two institutions, we do have here a set of representative responses from biomedical researchers who use human subjects.[14]

After describing in detail in Chapter 2 the design and methodology of our two studies, we proceed to report what we found, what the different patterns of expressed standards and self-reported behavior are with respect to the two key issues of informed consent and the risk-benefit ratio. The data, presented in Chapter 3, show two types of patterns. They show, first, that a majority of biomedical researchers using human subjects are very much aware of the importance of informed voluntary consent, that a majority express unwillingness to take undue risk when confronted with hypothetical research

---

[11] For only one of a great many statements of the absolute centrality of these two issues, see U.S. Department of Health, Education and Welfare—Public Health Service, *Protection of the Individual as a Research Subject* (Washington, D.C.: U.S. Government Printing Office, 1969), p. 8a. The problem of what constitutes "informed voluntary consent" is a complex one that deserves more theoretical and empirical attention than it has yet received. We hope to work on this problem in the near future. For some preliminary analyses by a variety of disciplinary specialists, see the *Daedalus* symposium, *op. cit.*, at pp. x, xii–xiii, 256, 284, 318ff., 323, 329, 345, 404, and 420 ff. In these pages we hear from physicians, lawyers, and sociologists. See also Lynn Chaiken Epstein and Louis Lasagna, "Obtaining Informed Consent: Form or Substance," *Archives of Internal Medicine*, 123 (1969): 682–88.

[12] This questionnaire can be found in Appendix I.

[13] This questionnaire can be found in Appendix II.

[14] The response rate of 72% includes 35 mailed questionaires received from researchers who refused a personal interview.

proposals, and that a majority do not themselves actually do studies in which the risk-benefit ratio is unfavorable for the patient-subjects. These patterns we call "strict." But the data also show that there is a significant minority that manifests a different type of pattern, what we call "more permissive," in each of these three respects: unawareness of the importance of, or concern with, consent; willingness to take undue risk; and actually doing studies that involve unfavorable risk-benefit ratios.

These two types of patterns, together with some other findings, are what the rest of our book seeks to explain. They are what we take as our dependent variables. Or rather, they are better seen as two "values" of each dependent variable, consisting of these ethical standards and behavior in this area of the use of human subjects for biomedical experimentation. One type of pattern is apparently the more "conforming" value of each variable, the other apparently the more "deviant" value of each variable. And both conformity and deviance with respect to each dependent variable, we feel, must be explained by the same independent variables, not by different variables.[15] It is variation in the same independent variables, we try to show, that does indeed help to explain the variation we find in each dependent variable.

Our explanations, or independent variables, are of two kinds. The first looks to the *conflict of equal values in socially structured situations* that puts pressure on some individuals to place one value ahead of another.[16] The second looks to three different types of *social control processes and structures*: socialization (or training) structures and processes, research collaboration groups and other informal interaction networks, and peer review committees.

Using our first kind of explanation, we assume that biomedical researchers face a conflict that we call "the dilemma of science and therapy" because they hold two equal but potentially conflicting values: to be an original discoverer in science and to be a physician who treats his patients humanely. As our data show, the majority of biomedical researchers are apparently in socially structured situations that permit them to balance these two values off against one another very nicely and thus to conform to both of them. But our data show that our more permissive or deviant researchers are in socially structured situations that put pressure on them to place the science value at least a little ahead of the humane therapy value. There are two of these so-

---

[15] For an excellent statement of the sociological theory of "social problems" and "deviant behavior," see Robert K. Merton, "Social Problems and Sociological Theory," in Robert K. Merton and Robert Nisbet, eds., *Contemporary Social Problems*, 3rd ed. (New York: Harcourt, Brace, Jovanovich, 1971).

[16] For a pioneer study focusing on value-conflict among biomedical innovators, see Renée C. Fox, *Experiment Perilous* (Glencoe, Ill.: The Free Press, 1959). See also another early study, Stewart E. Perry, *The Human Nature of Science* (New York: The Free Press, 1966).

cially structured situations that exert pressure toward deviance. One is the situation of *relative but deserved* failure in the structure of competition in the national and international biomedical research community. Here we have found that it is the "extreme mass producer," the man who publishes many papers that are not admired and therefore not cited by his scientific colleagues, who is more likely to manifest the more permissive patterns of ethical standards and behavior. The second situation is the one in which there occurs *relative but undeserved* failure to get just treatment in the structure of rewards in the local-institutional research setting. Here we have found that a more permissive pattern with respect to the risk-benefit ratios of his human studies is followed by the man who holds a less high rank in the local-institutional academic rank structure than his colleagues who have performed no more satisfactorily than he on any one of a number of criteria that are relevant for awarding rank in particular biomedical research institutions. Thus, two different types of social structure interact with a set of equal but potentially conflicting values, as social structures always interact with values to produce concrete behavioral outcomes, to produce the present patterns of conformity and deviance.

We turn next to our second kind of explanation, the processes and structures of social control. Our data show that the first type of social control, socialization, which is supposed to instill in researchers the knowledge, values, and norms necessary for satisfactory ethical performance with regard to the use of human subjects, is given scant attention in the formal medical school curriculum. Together with certain latent and informal socialization processes that are also occurring in medical school, this minimal concern in the formal curriculum results in only minimal effects on the more strict and the more permissive among our sample of biomedical researchers. Our data show that socialization into scientific values does occur in medical school but socializaton into humane treatment of human subjects has yet to be brought into its proper place in medical education.

The collaboration groups and other informal interaction networks in which our sample of biomedical researchers operate provide a second environment of social control for them in regard to standards and behavior in the treatment of human subjects. Our data show that like tends to select like for collaboration groups, that both the strict and the more permissive are more likely to work with their own kind, and that this collaboration of similars may contribute to deviance in groups where the more permissive predominate.

Finally, as is mandated by the National Institutes of Health for all the human research it subsidizes and as our data show is the case for all research in 85% of the institutions in our nationally representative sample, peer review committees exercise social control over biomedical research using human subjects. Our data show, both as measured by what the committees are reported to have actually done and by what our sample thinks about them, that the committees are fairly effective. For example, 31% of the institutions in our sample told us that some ethical revisions, but no rejections, have been required in research protocols; another 32% report one or more outright rejections; and, finally, 19% told us that there have been one or more instances where an investigator withdrew his proposal when he sensed that revision or rejection was likely. However, there is serious need for improvement in the use of the peer review committee as a control device. In our Intensive Two-Institution Study, for instance, 8% of our respondents *volunteered* the information that one or more of their investigations using human subjects had not come before the peer review committee, which, in each of the two institutions, apparently is supposed to review all research on humans.

So much by way of sociological explanation of the strict and more permissive patterns we have found. Based partly on our findings about these patterns of conformity and deviance, but also going beyond them on the basis of other knowledge we have about the nature of the professions and of social control processes, our final chapter asks some general questions about the social responsibilities of a powerful profession and makes some specific policy recommendations for reform in this area. Our general questions and our specific recommendations recognize that biomedical research is in considerable measure so esoteric an activity that a great deal of the social control that guides it must be in the hands of the biomedical research community itself. Yet, like all other specialized and esoteric social activities, biomedical research is too important to the larger society to be left entirely to its experts. In part it needs to be effectively and continuously scrutinized and controlled by outsiders. An effective system of control, including both insiders and outsiders, would better protect all the parties at interest, all the values, both science and humane therapy. As our society moves toward this system of more effective social control, we hope that the findings and analysis of this book will be of some assistance.

Before proceeding at last to the details of which we have just given a synoptic prospect, we wish to enter a few cautionary notes. We see at least two matters on which we want to warn against possible misunderstanding.

First, as progress is made in biomedical research, a number of different ethical problems arise, of which the proper treatment of human subjects in experimentation is *only one*. For example, even before the experimental phase in the development of a biomedical innovation is completed, but certainly thereafter, there often arise other ethical problems in connection with the allocation of scarce medical resources to those whose needs demand them. These ethical problems arise, for example, in such areas of tissue transplantation as kidney transplants (now "less experimental") and heart transplants (still "more experimental"). Such problems deserve research and analysis in their own right and are not attended to in this book.[17]

And second, we should like explicitly to disclaim having made any total explanation of the variations in the ethical standards and practices of bio-medical researchers using human subjects. There are almost certainly other cultural and social structural variables that help to determine ethical standards and practices than the ones we have used in this book. We hope that other research will soon supplement as well as refine our work. It is also very likely that psychological variables, which we have not dealt with at all, will turn out to be relevant to these expressed ethical standards and practices. Again, we hope that psychological research will soon supplement our work.

---

[17] For some excellent discussions of transplantation problems, see Renée C. Fox, "A Sociological Perspective on Organ Transplantation and Hemodialysis," in *Annals of the New York Academy of Sciences,* 169 (Jan. 21, 1970): 406–428, esp. at pp. 411–419 on allocation of scarce resources; and Roberta G. and Richard L. Simmons, "Organ Transplantation: A Societal Problem," *Social Problems,* 19(1971): 36–57. This article has an extensive bibliography. On the scientific and medical aspects of transplantation, see F. D. Moore, *Transplant: The Give and Take of Tissue Transplantation* (New York; Simon and Schuster, 1972).

For one fearful view of the problems involved in "genetic manipulation," see Leon R. Kass, "The New Biology: What Price Relieving Man's Estate?" *Science,* 174 (1971): 779–788.

2

RESEARCH DESIGN AND METHODOLOGY: THE TWO STUDIES

Our aim, as we indicated in the Introduction, was to collect valid, representative data on both the patterns and the social sources of conformity and deviance in researchers' expressed standards and actual behavior with regard to two key issues in the treatment of human research subjects: informed consent and the proper risk-benefit ratio. Given our analytic assumptions about some of the major sociological variables that might be relevant to our task, assumptions which will be spelled out in detail as we proceed with our analysis in later chapters, we needed to collect data on at least the following six matters:

1. The expressed standards and self-reported behavior of representative researchers using human subjects.

2. The formal characteristics of the institutions in which biomedical research is carried on.

3. Some standard sociological characteristics of our samples of researchers, together with data on the quantity and quality of their scientific work.

4. The patterns of socialization (or training) in the ethics of research using human subjects for our samples of researchers.

5. The structure and influence processes of the collaboration groups and various informal social networks in which biomedical researchers carry on their work.

6. The structure and processes of the formal peer review groups which have been mandated by the Public Health Service since 1966 and affect a considerable amount of American biomedical research.

To accomplish the rather large task just described, we chose to undertake two related but somewhat different kinds of study. In our first study, which we call National Survey, we attempted to collect some of our data from all of the institutions in the country in which biomedical research on human subjects is done. In our second study, which we call Intensive Two-Institution Study, we tried to interview all biomedical researchers engaged in studies using human subjects in two institutions chosen by cluster analysis to be representative of a very large number of the institutions in our National Survey sample. The important details about the methodology and execution of these two studies are given in the rest of this chapter. The questions we asked in these two studies can be examined in their entirety in Appendix I for National Survey and in Appendix II for Intensive Two-Institution Study. Details on how we used specific questions to provide important data are given as necessary in the rest of this chapter and in the later, more substantive and analytic chapters.

Besides our two studies, we collected important data from another source. To establish the scientific quality of an individual researcher's work, we used the *Science Citation Index*, an invaluable guide to work cited in the current scientific literature. Important details about the *Index* are provided in Chapter 4, where we make intensive use of it in our analysis.

NATIONAL SURVEY STUDY

The first problem needing solution before the national survey could be conducted was that of identifying the population of institutions in which biomedical research on humans is conducted. Since 1966, when the Public Health Service (P.H.S.) first announced its requirement that its grantee institutions in which research on humans is contemplated must submit an assurance of compliance with P.H.S. guidelines on the use of human subjects, the P.H.S. has maintained a cumulative list of institutions with acceptable assurances. On March 3, 1969, the list numbered about 1,600 institutions in the United States and some 130 acceptable foreign institutions. This list formed the base for our attempt to identify the relevant population of institutions for our study.

We were informed by representatives of the Division of Research Grants at P.H.S., however, that in many, if not most, of the institutions on the list, no biomedical research on humans was actually in progress. Large numbers of institutions submitted assurances to P.H.S. of their intent to comply with the guidelines if they ever engaged in any human research in the future. In another large number of institutions only non-biomedical (i.e., social or psychological) research on human subjects is done, and hence an assurance was submitted to cover that kind of research. Many institutions just seemed to want to express their generalized agreement with P.H.S. regulations by conforming to this specific regulation, even though it did not apply to them. The Division of Research Grants had no sublist of institutions in which biomedical research on humans is actually conducted, so various criteria had to be developed and applied to identify appropriate institutions from the master list.

We decided to be inclusive rather than exclusive in our attempt to pick out the right institutions from the list; that is, all borderline institutions would be sent a questionnaire. As a first step, we eliminated all colleges and universities at which there is no medical school, on the assumption that, among universities, only those with medical schools would have any *biomedical* research on humans. All prisons and reformatories were also eliminated. While research studies, often involving ethical problems, are done on prisoners, prisons and reformatories have no research staff that we might interview or who would be able to complete a questionnaire for us.[1] From the published studies it is apparent that a great deal of the research done in prisons is done by physicians affiliated with medical schools or teaching hospitals. Third, we specifically included all medical schools and hospitals, including mental hospitals. This left a large number of research institutions whose eligibility still had to be determined, however. The research institutes were looked up in the *Research Centers Directory* to see if any studies involving humans were explicitly listed or whether the *Directory* mentioned explicitly that studies involving human subjects were not done. This clarified many cases, and any remaining institutions whose status was still not clear were included in the research population.

There remained, however, one essential problem with our list: we could not be certain that all institutions in which we were interested had indeed submitted assurances to P.H.S., thus placing their names on our list. For example, institutions in which human research is funded only through non-P.H.S. sources would not have to submit an assurance to P.H.S. Also, some institutions were just slow in complying, and over the three-year period between the first issuance of the guidelines in 1966 and the publishing of our list in March 1969, the number of assurances had risen dramatically. But it might not yet be absolutely complete.

We know, however, that N.I.H. supplies about 35% of all funds for support of medical research in this country.[2] No institution with even a small research program could afford not to seek as much money as possible from that source. Thus, the likelihood that any major research institution is totally non-P.H.S. funded is very small. We could assume, then, with considerable

---

[1] For some interesting analysis and empirical data on the use of prisoners as research subjects, see John D. Arnold, Daniel C. Martin, and Sarah E. Boyer, "A Study of One Prison Population and Its Response to Medical Research," in Irving Ladimer, ed., *New Dimensions in Legal and Ethical Concepts for Human Research*, in *Annals of the New York Academy of Sciences*, 169 (Jan. 21, 1970), Art. 2: pp. 463–470; Daniel C. Martin, John D. Arnold, R. F. Zimmerman, and Robert H. Richart, "Human Subjects in Clinical Research—A Report of Three Studies," *New England Journal of Medicine*, 279 (1968): 1426–1431; and Kenneth G. Kohlstaedt, "Conducting Investigational Drug Studies for Industry," in Ladimer, ed., *op. cit.*, pp. 496–502.

[2] National Institutes of Health, *Basic Data for 1968* (Washington, D.C.: U.S. Government Printing Office, 1968), p. 5.

confidence, that very few major institutions of the type we wanted to study were not on the P.H.S. list of assurances by 1969. As a further check, we examined the *Research Centers Directory* carefully for institutions in which biomedical research on humans is done that were not on the P.H.S. list. We discovered nine such institutions and included them in our population. The total number of institutions in our population after all the above procedures were carried out came to 681. We hoped that any institutions in this very inclusive group in which we did not really need to be interested would become known to us through their responses to certain questionnaire items. In addition, however, we planned a short follow-up questionnaire of nonrespondents both to further clarify which institutions would form the final population and to provide us with data for a nonresponse analysis.

Our questionnaire was sent on May 26, 1969 to the individual in each institution with whom P.H.S. negotiated that institution's assurance of compliance. Sometimes this person was merely an administrative contracting officer who was not really familiar with the research situation, and he then referred the questionnaire to a person in the organization who could better answer the questions. In larger organizations this referral process sometimes went through more than one step, and consequently we decided to allow plenty of time for our respondents to complete the questionnaire. December 1 was, therefore, set as the cutoff date, and questionnaires received after that date were not to be included in our analysis. As it turned out, none were received after cutoff.

Our respondent-individuals were fairly typical of active researchers and those who participate in the peer review process. In 87% of the cases our eventual respondent was a member of the institution's committee to review research proposals contemplating the use of human subjects, and 72% were researchers who use humans as subjects in their studies. To obtain information about the expressed standards of this set of people on the ethical issues involved in biomedical research on humans, we included six hypothetical research proposals for the individual respondent's review in which ethical dilemmas of various kinds were presented. Ideas about what specific hypothetical proposals would best suit our purposes came from two sources: our own reading of the medical literature and from various persons who are concerned with the problems we were addressing in our studies. We then wrote eight possible hypothetical proposals and submitted them to a distinguished biomedical researcher for his comments and suggestions. He helped us refine four of them, made us eliminate four as unsuited to our purposes and then suggested and helped us write two new hypothetical proposals.[3] These six pro-

---

[3] These six hypotheticals can be examined in Appendix I and will be presented in detail in the next and some succeeding chapters.

posals were refined and presented, in pre-test interviews, to a total of 11 researchers at nine institutions who were asked for their comments and criticisms in light of the purposes the questions were supposed to serve. We were concerned that the hypothetical proposals be short, concise, and accurate, yet include enough information to allow our respondents to think of them as real research proposals. On two or three of the questions our pretest interviewees discovered and corrected factual errors for us. On two occasions they pointed out errors but could not give us the right information, and so referred us to a distinguished man in the scientific field in which we had made an error. All of the hypothetical proposals, as it turned out, were either studies already published or studies in progress in at least one institution in the country. They are, then, "hypothetical-actual," not "hypothetical-fantastic."

Some questions were intended to ascertain the individual's social background, and some his actual experiences. The analysis of the responses of these individuals was intended as exploratory only, of course, since we expected that the sample of individual respondents we would get from our national survey was very likely to be somewhat biased in favor of senior people. After four mailed follow-ups and a scattering of telephone conversations, 302 completed questionnaires were returned. Nine of the questionnaires were completely filled out but the answers clearly indicated that at that time no biomedical research on humans was being done at the institutions. Since the respondents in these nine institutions were all physicians, the information on the questionnaires was used in our analysis of the respondents as persons, but the institutions were dropped from the population of institutions, making the total response 293 institutions. Many letters were received from other institutions informing us that no biomedical research on humans was actually done at the institution, even though an assurance was submitted to P.H.S. Reasons why this might occur were outlined earlier. In addition, we sent to all nonrespondents a one-page follow-up questionnaire in which we specifically asked whether biomedical research on humans was performed in the institution. Three questions about the functions, number of researchers, and productivity[4] of the researchers at the institutions were also asked so that we could compare respondents with nonrespondents on those items.

Seventy-five of these one-page questionnaires were returned from institutions where biomedical research on humans is done. Another 158 institutions were excluded from the population because their representatives informed us, either by letter or by answering "no" to the relevant question of the one-page questionnaire, that no biomedical research on humans is done

---

[4] Institutional productivity was measured by asking the respondent to report the approximate number of scientific papers based on work using human subjects published by researchers in the institutions for 1968.

at their institutions. The remaining 155 institutions either refused by letter or did not respond at all to anything. All of these were classified, of course, as nonrespondents. The final population, then, was made up of 523 institutions and 293 of them sent us completed, usable questionnaires for a response rate of 56%.

When respondents were compared with nonrespondents on the items for which comparison was possible, there were some differences. Medical schools responded slightly more often than the population as a whole, and mental hospitals responded much more often than the population as a whole (see Table 2.1). The "other" category in Table 2.1 is populated largely with

Table 2.1. Respondents by Type of Institution

	Medical Schools	Teach. Hosp. Affil. with Med. School	Mental Hosp.	Other	Total
Respondent	64%	59%	74%	42%	56%
Nonrespondent	36	41	26	58	44
Totals	100% (92) 18%	100% (97) 19%	100% (110) 21%	100% (224) 43%	100% (523) 100%

teaching hospitals not affiliated with any medical school, small general hospitals, research institutes, and other smaller institutions. They responded less often than the population as a whole.

It must be pointed out that the low population size for "teaching hospitals affiliated with medical schools" is due to the fact that many medical schools included their teaching hospitals under a blanket assurance to P.H.S., and hence all the teaching hospitals did not appear in our list of separate assurances. When this was the case, some of our respondents included their teaching hospitals in their answers to our questionnaire. We knew about this problem in advance and could have obtained a list of all hospitals affiliated with accredited medical schools from the annual bulletin of the American Association of Medical Colleges. The problems in this approach, however, would have been much greater than those inherent in the approach we chose. Many medical schools list as affiliated hospitals all their endowed "hospitals," named for a benefactor but having no administrative apparatus separate from the medical school or the overall university hospital. Had we sent questionnaires to all teaching hospitals, then, we would have included in our population many nonexistent institutions, artificially inflating the population size.

We received direct responses from 59 medical schools, but the research of some of the faculty of 15 more medical schools is represented in our sample by a questionnaire from one or more of their affiliated teaching hospitals. Ninety-two medical schools appear in our overall population, 14 short of the population of 106 known medical schools in 1968. This is because 7 medical schools wrote to us that no biomedical research on humans is done on their campuses and because 7 more schools were still in such an early stage of development that we decided not to contact them.

Institutions that identify with a religious grouping, either through sponsorship or direct control,[5] were no more or less likely to respond to our questionnaire, and highly productive research institutions were no more or less likely to respond. Institutions with higher numbers of clinical researchers tended to respond slightly more often than those with fewer researchers.

The response rate by type of institution tells us what types of institutions were more or less motivated to respond to our questionnaire, but more crucial for determining the representativeness of our response is the question of the representativeness of individual institutions within a type, for example whether those medical schools that did respond were different in any way from those who did not respond. Among medical schools and teaching hospitals affiliated with medical schools, those who responded were no more or less likely to be highly productive or heavily involved in research as indicated by the number of people engaged in clinical research. Among mental hospitals, highly productive institutions responded slightly more often, but the difference was not significant. Mental hospitals with a large number of researchers responded significantly more often, however. In our "other" category, which was made up mostly of teaching hospitals not affiliated with a medical school, community general hospitals, and research institutes, there were no differences between respondents and nonrespondents on the above items.

We can say, then, that our data are representative of medical schools, of their affiliated teaching hospitals, and of those institutions in our "other" category, at least on productivity and number of clinical researchers. Our data underrepresent less productive mental hospitals that have few researchers. This underrepresentation means only that the institutions that did respond represent a slightly higher proportion of the biomedical research on humans that is being done in mental hospitals than the proportion of respondents would indicate. That sort of bias can be viewed as beneficial in a study such as ours.

---

[5] We asked for religious affiliation, if any, on our large questionnaire, and obtained this information for nonrespondents from a number of different sources. Sometimes the affiliation was printed on the institution's letterhead, so if we had correspondence from an institution we sometimes obtained the information that way. Many times we used the name of the institution as an indicator. The data on religious affiliation, then, is less reliable than that for other items.

INTENSIVE TWO-INSTITUTION STUDY

In our second study we wanted very much to interview a set of biomedical researchers that was in some sense representative of all biomedical researchers whose work involves human subjects. That was desirable so that we could check some of the findings from our analysis of the individuals who responded to our National Survey. A national probability sample of researchers might seem best for this purpose. In order to study intercolleague influence as a mechanism of social control, however, a national probability sample of researchers, while ideal for obtaining a representative sample of researchers, could not reliably provide us with data on researchers who collaborate or otherwise associate *in person* with each other. We decided, therefore, to construct a typology of institutions in which biomedical research on humans is conducted using data from our first study and to interview all of the clinical researchers in one institution from each type. In this way we could be fairly sure that the full range of researchers and research would be represented in an interview population of manageable size. In addition, since most researchers could be expected to collaborate with others in their institutions, this strategy would allow us the chance to interview all of the collaborators on many research projects, which is of course essential in studying intercolleague influence. Such a population, it turns out, would also be an acceptable one for our study of formal and informal socialization and their effects on the formation of ethical standards and behavior.

To construct a typology of the institutions in our National Survey, we decided to use cluster analysis. Cluster analysis is a method of identifying sets of characteristics that are highly correlated with each other but not with the rest of some larger set of characteristics. Louis L. McQuitty[6] describes a very simple cluster analysis technique called elementary linkage analysis which can be completed in a short time by hand. McQuitty's examples, however, involve the use of various correlation coefficients that are applicable only to variables which are at least ordinal, and some of ours are nominal. In the dichotomous case, however, nominal and ordinal variates look the same so we decided to dichotomize all of our variates if possible and use the Tau B statistic. Tau B, though it assumes ordinality, does not assume anything about the causal direction of the relationship between two variables. It is a symmetric statistic.

From our National Survey data twenty institutional-level variables were available for elementary linkage analysis. Mental hospitals were excluded from consideration because we had discovered that most mental hospitals do

---

[6] "Elementary Linkage Analysis for Isolating Orthogonal and Oblique Types . . . ," *Educational and Psychological Measurement*, 17, no. 2 (1957): 207–229.

little research of the type in which we are interested, and to go through all of the trouble to obtain access to one of them would not reward us with many interviews. Institutions with large numbers of mental patients which did not identify themselves as mental hospitals were included, and they formed a separate cluster, as we shall see shortly. The twenty variables involved in the analysis are described in Table 2.2, and the Tau B matrix and the resultant clusters appear in Table 2.3. Note that variable 37 is a trichotomous variable. Type of institution could not be meaningfully dichotomized, and so the categories were placed in the order in which they affect the other variables in the matrix. This order was the same in all cases.

Five clusters of variables result from applying elementary linkage analysis to our Tau B matrix. Three clusters can be excluded from consideration because they are substantially trivial. Cluster II, for example, merely indicates that institutions with a large proportion of lower-class patients also have a large proportion of lower-class research subjects. Clusters IV and V are similar to Cluster II in that they show that institutions with a high proportion of children or terminal patients also have high proportions of children or terminal patients as subjects.

The remaining two clusters, I and III, are meaningful, however. Cluster I is a cluster of four variables centered around public institutions that have high proportions of older and mental patients. The high end of this group is made up of the institutions which most resemble mental hospitals but which do not call themselves mental hospitals. We decided that we were not interested in comparing the two types resulting from this cluster for the same reason mental hospitals were excluded from consideration at the outset.

That leaves us with Cluster III, which shows that institutions with a large number of researchers are much more likely to be: highly productive; those with a large research budget; medical schools or teaching hospitals closely affiliated with medical schools; institutions that strongly encourage research; institutions doing research that is risky for the human subjects involved; institutions doing research at the scientific frontier; and institutions receiving a high proportion of their research money from the Public Health Service.

In order to learn something about biomedical research institutions that are at different points along the organizational dimension represented by Cluster III, we decided to examine an institution that is fairly high on all of the correlated variables making up Cluster III and one that is fairly low. The high group of institutions can be represented very well by almost any university hospital and research center. Small community teaching hospitals not affiliated with a medical school were the most numerous institutions in the low group of institutions in the cluster. While this kind of choice in no way assures us that our interviewees are representative of the population of bio-

Table 2.2. Variables Used in the Cluster Analysis

Variable   3: Is the Institution Public or Private?
Public; Private

Variable 528: Proportion of Subjects Who Are Mental Patients
Low = 0–10%; High = More Than 10%

Variable 527: Proportion of Subjects Who Are Older People
Low = 0–15%; High = More Than 15%

Variable 507: Proportion of Patients Who Are Mental Patients
Low = 0–10%; High = More Than 10%

Variable 504: Proportion of Patients Who Are Lower Class
Low = 0–35%; High = More Than 35%

Variable 525: Proportion of Research Subjects Who Are Lower Class
Low= 0–35%; High = More Than 35%

Variable 46: Proportion of Clinical Research in the Institution Which Involves Moderate or High Risk for the Subjects
Zero; Any

Variable 17: Size of the Research Budget
Low = Zero to $500,000; High = More Than $500,000

Variable 19: Number of Clinical Researchers
Low = 0–25 Researchers; High = More Than 25 Researchers

Variable 11: Number of Clinical Research Papers Published by the Researchers in the Institution in 1968
Low = 0–10 Papers; High = More Than 10 Papers

Variable   8: Degree Institution Encourages Research
Strongly Encourages; Moderately or Does Not Encourage

Variable 37: Type of Institution
Medical School; Teaching Hospital Affiliated With a Medical School; Other

Variable   9: Is Any Research of the Frontier Type Done in the Institution?
Yes; No

Variable 18: Proportion of Research Money From PHS
High = Three-Fourths or More; Low = Less Than Three-Fourths

Variable 506: Proportion of Patients Who Are Older People
Low = 0–25%; High = More Than 25%

Variable 505: Proportion of Patients Who Are Children
Low = 0–8%; High = More Than 8%

Variable 526: Proportion of Subjects Who Are Children
Low = 0–5%; High = More Than 5%

Variable 508: Proportion of Patients Who Are Terminal
Low = 0–3%; High = More Than 3%

Variable 529: Proportion of Subjects Who Are Terminal
Low = Zero; High = Any

Variable 10: Proportion of Researchers Who Work Alone
High = Three-Fourths or More; Low = Less Than Three-Fourths

---

medical researchers using human subjects, we felt that learning about research done at a less high-powered institution might at least place our findings a bit more in perspective. It was our feeling that the treatment of human subjects of research would be less adequate at a high-powered institution, such as a university hospital, where researchers are under more pressure to produce published scientific work, and we did not want to generalize to biomedical research as a whole after examining only that type of institution.

We decided that the university hospital and research center selected should have a good reputation and that its researchers should not, as a population, be markedly different from the average as far as social background is concerned. We were less concerned about the community teaching hospital not affiliated with a medical school because we expected fewer than 50 interviews from it out of a total population of about 400 expected interviews.

The university hospital and research center that was finally chosen for intensive analysis was, then, of high quality and large size, with a population of clinical researchers that, as a group, was relatively heterogeneous in the social background of its members.[7] In the selection of the community and teaching hospital not affiliated with a medical school, however, we ran into some practical problems. We wanted to obtain sufficient interviews from our "low-speed" institution to characterize it by some aggregate statistics. The cutoff point on "number of researchers" in order to be called "large" in our cluster analysis was just 25 researchers. We felt that we would need at least 40 in order to characterize the institution using aggregate statistics. We finally selected a community and teaching hospital with about 70 clinical researchers so that we could be sure of getting 40 to 50 interviews after refusals. The university hospital and research center we selected reported about 520 clinical researchers in its questionnaire response. In addition, researchers at the community and teaching hospital produce about 50 papers involving human subjects each year, well over the lower cutoff point of 10 papers for the high category on productivity. The researchers at the university hospital and research center, however, produced over 850 papers reporting such research involving human subjects in 1969 according to their annual report. The two institutions clearly represent opposite types in terms of size, even though the community and teaching hospital falls a bit above our cutoff for both productivity and number of clinical researchers.

Early analysis of our interview responses provided some further confirmation that our choice of institutions did provide the sort of contrast of

---

[7] Our University Hospital and Research Center is very much like the one described in Emily Mumford, *Interns: From Students to Physicians* (Cambridge, Mass.: Harvard University Press, 1970). However, our Community and Teaching Hospital is not like her community hospital, which is apparently not at all involved in research.

Table 2.3. Tau B Coefficient Matrix for Elementary Linkage Analysis

Variable Numbers	Variable Numbers																			
	3	528	527	507	504	525	46	17	19	11	8	37	9	18	506	505	526	508	529	10
3		.37	.30	.32	.33	.23	.21	.17	.18	.05	.18	.18	.04	.02	.02	.03	.02	.13	.06	.04
528	.37		.91	.74	.08	.15	.14	.06	.07	.09	.12	.10	.12	.00	.10	.03	.07	.06	.02	.02
527	.30	.91		.71	.08	.17	.07	.00	.01	.04	.14	.09	.05	.04	.13	.09	.03	.16	.01	.04
507	.32	.74	.71		.05	.13	.17	.08	.03	.07	.11	.11	.05	.04	.11	.02	.06	.11	.04	.06
504	.33	.08	.05	.05		.76	.09	.15	.08	.13	.07	.12	.12	.12	.02	.05	.03	.14	.09	.04
525	.23	.15	.17	.13	.76		.02	.05	.10	.01	.13	.01	.02	.04	.01	.06	.07	.00	.00	.17
46	.21	.14	.07	.09	.02	.02		.24	.39	.35	.05	.25	.20	.15	.03	.19	.09	.26	.37	.07
17	.17	.06	.00	.08	.15	.05	.24		.52	.42	.20	.36	.24	.19	.14	.10	.12	.14	.11	.14
19	.18	.07	.01	.03	.08	.10	.39	.52		.52	.22	.42	.24	.21	.02	.06	.01	.18	.24	.17
11	.05	.09	.04	.07	.13	.01	.35	.42	.52		.19	.22	.35	.30	.14	.05	.07	.03	.06	.17
8	.18	.12	.14	.11	.07	.13	.05	.20	.22	.19		.12	.16	.04	.05	.07	.09	.06	.05	.05
37	.18	.10	.09	.11	.12	.01	.25	.36	.42	.35	.12		.16	.14	.21	.10	.10	.03	.18	.21
9	.04	.12	.05	.05	.12	.02	.20	.24	.24	.35	.16	.16		.20	.04	.10	.11	.25	.16	.17
18	.02	.00	.04	.04	.12	.04	.15	.19	.21	.30	.04	.14	.20		.05	.02	.06	.03	.03	.07

Table 2.3 (*cont.*)

506	.02	.10	.13	.11	.02	.01	.03	.14	.02	.05	.05	.10	.04	.05	.28	.23	.22	.16	.13
505	.03	.03	.09	.02	.05	.06	.19	.10	.06	.07	.07	.10	.10	.02	.28	.51	.01	.03	.10
526	.02	.07	.03	.06	.03	.07	.09	.12	.01	.03	.09	.03	.11	.06	.23	.51	.01	.03	.01
508	.13	.06	.16	.11	.14	.00	.26	.14	.13	.18	.06	.18	.25	.03	.22	.01	.01	.37	.09
529	.06	.02	.01	.04	.09	.00	.37	.11	.24	.27	.05	.21	.16	.03	.16	.03	.03	.37	.09
10	.04	.02	.04	.06	.04	.17	.07	.14	.17	.17	.05	.11	.17	.07	.13	.10	.01	.09	.09

Cluster I

```
       507
3 ———— 528 ═══ 527
```

Cluster II

```
504 ═══ 525
```

Cluster III

```
        17 ——— 46
         ‖
8 ——— 19 ═══ 11 ——— 9
         |
        37 ——— 18
```

Cluster IV

```
506
 |
505 ═══ 526
```

Cluster V

```
508 ═══ 529
```

types revealed by the cluster. Interviewees from both institutions were engaged in about the same number of research projects per person, on the average, but those at the university hospital and research center are notably more likely to spend more than three-fifths of their time doing research, 29%(321) versus 15%(54). They were also much more likely to view their institution as strongly pressuring them to do research, 36%(281) versus 18%(45). In addition, at the community and teaching hospital, fully 61%(69) of the research projects involving humans that were being conducted at the time we were interviewing involved no risk whatsoever to the human subjects while that was true in only 41% (353) of the studies at the University hospital and research center. Finally, although the differences involved are smaller, the biomedical researchers at the University hospital and research center had more frequently published more than ten papers in the past five years, 36%(320) versus 30%(54); and also their publications more often had received more than seven citations in their three most highly cited years, according to a count using the *Science Citation Index*.[8]

Once we selected the two institutions whose clinical researchers we wished to interview, there remained the problems of identifying the subpopulation of researchers who engage in research on human subjects and arranging interviews with them. Both institutions, as is common among research institutions, publish an annual report that contains a bibliography of all staff publications. In the case of our two institutions the title of the paper very often indicated whether or not human subjects had been involved in the study. We could then compile a list of researchers by recording the authors and co-authors of all papers that seemed to involve human subjects. In addition, both annual reports included sections where each department summarized the previous year's activities, including the kind of research that was going on and who the researchers were.

In order to identify researchers involved in studies on humans who did not appear in either the bibliography or the annual report and to discover who was working with whom, we planned to ask each interviewee who his collaborators were. Using the initial list as a large base we could, then, initiate a "snowball sample" once we started interviewing. Since the initial sample, based on the bibliography and the annual report, would be quite large, it would be unlikely that many researchers in whom we were interested would not be in it. The snowball technique would fill in the small number of gaps. In addition, once we began making personal contact with prospective respondents we could eliminate from the list any who could convince us that they were not engaged in any human research.

---

[8] For full details on the *Science Citation Index* and the significance of such citation counts for scientific quality, see Chapter 4.

Having worked out a way of generating a population of researchers, we then faced the problem of access, often a difficult problem for social researchers. We made an appointment to discuss the study with a high administrative officer in each institution to inform him of our intention to study his institution and to make sure that he would not object. We explained the study to each officer in some detail and informed him that we intended to contact his researchers independently, without official approval, leaving it up to each individual researcher to cooperate with us or not as he himself saw fit. The study would be explained to each researcher in a cover letter, and no mention of institutional approval or disapproval would be made. We would assure each researcher that his name, those of his colleagues, and that of his institution would be kept strictly confidential. This approach proved to be acceptable to the researchers we contacted as is evident in their response; only one interviewee asked us if we had obtained official approval. He agreed to be interviewed only after he cleared it with the administrator with whom we had talked.

The interviewing took place over a period of six months, from January to June 1970. Because of the complexity of the issues being studied and the high status of our interviewees, all interviews were conducted by members of our immediate research group, with the help of two full-time, highly competent interviewers. A total of 950 potential respondents were eventually contacted by letter, including "snowballs," 78 at the community and teaching hospital and 872 at the university hospital and research center, and as many as ten telephone follow-ups were made in an individual case in order to schedule interviews. Some 411 of those contacted turned out to be engaged only in test-tube research, animal research, or no research at all and were eliminated from the population. By the end of June 352 interviews had been completed which averaged about 1½ to 2 hours in length. Fifty-four were completed at the community and teaching hospital and 298 at the university hospital and research center. A total of 187 of those researchers contacted were classified as refusals at that time.

The first four or five interviews, all at the community and teaching hospital, served as a pre-test of the interview schedule.[9] Since many of the ques-

---

[9] See Appendix II for this interview schedule. Specific questions will be discussed as necessary in later chapters. We should also note here, and we will explain more fully later, that a change was made in the list of hypothetical proposals from the National Survey questionnaire to the Intensive Two-Institution interview schedule. Because our mail respondents had indicated the great length of time it took them to respond to the six hypotheticals in their questionnaire, and because we knew how limited our time would be in the personal interviews with the busy researchers in our second study, we shortened the list of hypotheticals from six to two and changed the second of these two slightly to make sure we got separate responses for the informed consent and the risk-benefit ratio

tions had been asked of the respondents to the national survey study, the interview schedule went smoothly from the start. At weekly meetings of our research group the interviewing was discussed extensively in order to be sure that we were all interviewing in as uniform a manner as possible. In an analysis of interviewer effects which we completed as soon as the data were ready for machine processing, no significant differences were found on any of our questions in the responses of researchers who were interviewed by one member of our group as opposed to any of the others.

In addition to data on our interviewees, data on 424 research projects involving human subjects were obtained from our 352 interviews. Sociograms showing the collaborating researchers were drawn for each project. In only about half of the projects, however, had all collaborators been interviewed. It was decided at that point that one final attempt would be made to obtain data from prior refusals so that in more instances we might have data on all collaborators in a project. A shortened questionnaire containing the most important items and requesting a mailed response was, therefore, sent to the 187 refusals. Of this group 35 completed the questionnaire after one mailed follow-up, all but two of them from the university hospital and research center. Thus, we had either an interview or a mailed questionnaire response from 331 researchers at the university hospital and research center and from 56 researchers at the community and teaching hospital. The final total of refusals was 152.

Our total response, then, was 387 researchers interviewed or characterized by questionnaire out of 539 eligible, or 72%. Of these 387, 66 researchers were between projects on humans when we interviewed them. They were in the process of planning new research, and many were involved in projects using animals. Most of our analysis in later chapters deals only with the 312 researchers who said that they were involved in a project involving human subjects at the time we interviewed them. These researchers provided data for us on 424 research projects involving human subjects, and in 227 of the projects (54%) all collaborators were interviewed or completed the mailed questionnaire.

Although most of those contacted who refused to be interviewed insisted that they were only peripherally involved in research with humans or that they were too busy to take the time for our study, we made an attempt to discover whether there were any systematic differences between respondents and nonrespondents. For those nonrespondents who were listed in the annual publication of their respective institutions we obtained information

---

issues. (Our actual interview experience justified our fears and the change we based on them.) The two hypotheticals can be examined in Appendix II and compared with the six in Appendix I. We will compare them in detail in the next chapter.

about their rank, either academic or professional. Only those at University hospital and research center, of course, had academic rank. As Table 2.4

Table 2.4. Comparison of the Academic and Professional Ranks of Respondents and Nonrespondents

Academic Rank	Resp.	Nonresp.	Professional Rank	Resp.	Nonresp.
Professor	23%	22%	Consultant	2%	2%
Assoc. Prof.	22	30	Attending	18	21
Asst. Prof.	34	30	Assoc. Att.	18	17
Other	21	17	Att. Att.	33	28
			Other	30	31
	100%	100%		100%	100%
	(222)	(121)		(326)	(131)

indicates, the distribution of rank, both professional and academic, is similar for respondents and for those nonrespondents for whom we could obtain this information. There was also no difference in the proportion of respondents and nonrespondents who were physicians, dentists, and other nonphysicians. We also compared those projects in which all members had been interviewed with those in which some investigators identified as working on those projects had refused to be interviewed. The incomplete projects did not seem, in general, to involve more serious risks. On the basis of these data, then, we can find no systematic differences between the respondents and the nonrespondents which would affect our findings.

Because there are few if any precedents for the research on experimenting with humans that we are reporting in this book, we have reported our research design and methodology with particular care. As they become necessary and relevant, still further details are provided in later chapters. But enough has now been done to permit us to move to more substantive and analytic matters. In the next chapter we report what our data show about current standards and practices in this area. We hope to be able to provide an answer to the implicit question that informs much discussion on the subject. Is there a problem? In later chapters we try to account for the patterns of conformity and deviance that current standards and practices reveal.

3

IS THERE A PROBLEM? CURRENT PATTERNS OF ETHICAL STANDARDS AND PRACTICES

In the Introduction we stated that the data from our two studies, National Survey and Intensive Two-Institution Study, reveal two patterns in the ethical standards and practices of biomedical researchers. There is a conforming pattern and a deviant pattern or, perhaps better, there is a "strict" pattern and a "more permissive" pattern. The fact that the more permissive pattern exists suggests that there is indeed a problem in this area, that the increased concern shown by both the biomedical research community itself and the lay community over ethical standards of researchers whose studies use human subjects is not without some objective basis. In this chapter we present the details on the data and analysis from which we established the existence of these two patterns.

As noted in the previous chapter, in our National Survey we asked the person who responded for his institution to evaluate six hypothetical research proposals in which ethical dilemmas were presented.[1] In the two-institution study, only two of the hypothetical proposals from the national study were again presented, and one of these was slightly different from its earlier form. (Our reasons for this decision were presented in footnote 9, Ch. 2.)

The two proposals chosen for the second study were ones for which there had been a good distribution of approvals and disapprovals in our National Survey. We hoped for a similar distribution of responses to the two questions in our interview study so that there would be enough cases available for analysis if we wished to compare extreme types or control for the effects of other factors. Thus, an analysis of the responses to these two sets of hypothetical proposals will give us some idea of the expressed ethical standards of our two groups of respondents.

In the second study, of course, we also gathered data on the several human studies in which our respondents were then engaged.[2] For each of these

---

[1] See the previous chapter for a description of how the proposals were developed, and see Appendix I for a copy of the questionnaire.

[2] See questions 3H, 3I, 3J, and 3K in our interview schedule (Appendix II).

studies, we have our interviewees' estimates of the risks to the subjects involved, the hoped-for benefits for present subjects and for future patients, and interviewees' estimates of the importance of the scientific knowledge to be gained. An analysis of these data will allow us to describe the actual ethical practices of our respondents and to see how their practices are related to their expressed ethical standards.

The use of self-reported data on conforming and deviant behavior is a risky business insofar as the respondents may underreport the amount of deviance. In the case of our research, since the consequences of error for policy recommendations would be great, caution is necessary in the interpretation of the sort of questions we asked. On the other hand, however, we can be quite sure that our respondents are not likely to have tried to make themselves and medical research look worse than it actually is. The number of respondents whose ethical standards and practices are ranged on the permissive end of our scales is likely, if anything, to be an underestimate of the actual amount of permissiveness.

It must be remembered throughout that the populations surveyed in our two studies are somewhat different in their social composition. Respondents who were clinical researchers and/or physicians in our first study tended, on the whole, to be more senior. This was because the names we obtained from the Public Health Service were senior institutional representatives with whom P.H.S. had negotiated institutional assurances. Our second study was intended to be a more representative sample, and hence there were many more junior researchers in that group. The bias toward senior people in our National Survey is actually a bonus in at least one way, however. If evidence for concern can be presented about the ethical standards of a group of senior and influential clinical researchers and physicians, 87% of whom serve on their institution's research review committee, as is the case in our national study, it should certainly carry more weight than evidence from a sample which is biased in the opposite direction or from even a representative sample. That is so because senior researchers and physicians can be expected to have a greater influence on the quality of ethical norms in biomedical research, especially as a result of decisions they make in their capacity as members of institutional review committees.

Because our two groups of respondents do differ in their social composition, a brief comparative summary of the characteristics of each group is necessary. In our National Survey not all respondents were clinical researchers or physicians, since some institutions designated an administrator to complete our questionnaire. In our intensive interview study all respondents were either presently engaged in a study involving human subjects or had been so engaged within the past two years. For our comparison and subsequent analysis, then, only respondents from the National Survey who were, either researchers presently engaged in a human study or were physicians not presently engaged in a human study are included. The total number of individuals available for this analysis from our national study is 260 out of the 293 respondents.

First our National Survey respondents are older than those in our Intensive Two-Institution Study (see Table 3.1).

Table 3.1 Age of Respondents to Our Two Studies

Age	National Survey	Intensive Two-Institution Study
26–35	8%	36%
36–45	38	38
46 or older	54	26
	100% (254)	100% (380)

Second, the respondents from our Two-Institution Study were more productive in the last five years than those from our National Survey. Of the respondents in our second study 49% produced more than seven scientific papers in the last five years, while only 38% of the respondents in our National Survey did so. We thought this might be because older researchers have been found, in our first study and in other studies,[3] to produce fewer papers per year, and our first study had an older group of respondents. When we compared the productivity of the researchers in the two studies controlling for age, we found no difference in productivity for those under 45 for the two samples but large differences in the over-45 age group. The older researchers in our interview study were more than twice as likely (67% to 31%) to have produced more than seven scientific papers in the last five years.

Conversely, however, only 27% of the respondents in our Intensive Two-Institution Study received more than seven citations to the total number of papers they published in their three most heavily cited years, while 41% of the respondents in our National Survey received more than seven citations.[4] If the number of citations is used as a measure of quality of the re-

---

[3] Wayne Dennis, "Age and Productivity Among Scientists," *Science,* 123 (n.d.): 724–25. For a later and subtler analysis of this problem, see Harriet Zuckerman and Robert K. Merton, "Age, Aging and Age Structure in Science," in Matilda White Riley, Marilyn Johnson, and Anne Foner, *Aging and Society,* Vol. III (New York: Russell Sage Foundation, 1972).

[4] The decision to use the total number of citations to all the work in the respondent's three most highly cited years is based on work reported in Stephen Cole and Jonathan

search, or of the utility of his work for other researchers, this means that respondents to our National Survey were of higher average quality. When we compared the number of citations received by our respondents in the two studies controlling for age, those under 45 in the National Survey were twice as likely (44% to 22%) to have more than seven citations. Researchers in the over-45 group were equally likely to have more than seven citations when the respondents in the two studies are compared. Combining inferences from our analyses of productivity and citations, we can see that respondents to our National Survey questionnaire received more citations in proportion to papers produced in the last five years, on the average, than did respondents in our Intensive Two-Institution Study.

Third, there was a higher proportion of Protestants in our National Survey. Table 3.2 compares the two samples on religion. There was absolutely zero difference between the two samples on religiousness, however. We asked respondents in both studies the following question: "Do you consider yourself deeply religious? moderately religious? largely indifferent to religion? basically opposed to religion?" In both studies 53% of the respondents indicated that they are "deeply or moderately" religious. Since our analysis shows ethical standards and practices not to be different by religious affiliation, the difference between our two samples in this area is not important.

Fourth and last, the respondents to our intensive interview study were more liberal politically than respondents to our national study. Of the respondents in our second study 52% were political liberals while only 39% of those in our National Survey were.

R. Cole, "Scientific Output and Recognition," *American Sociological Review*, 32, no. 3 (1967): 380. The Coles state that "it is possible that the total number of citations to a man's work is not a completely independent indicator of quality, since scientists who publish a large number of papers each of which receives only a few citations might accumulate as many citations as those who have published only a few papers which are heavily cited." They "therefore decided to take the number of citations to the three most heavily cited contributions by each physicist as an indicator of the impact of his best work. Since a contribution in physics does not typically take the form of a single paper, but is usually presented in a series of papers, we have used citations to the year's output rather than the single paper as our unit of measure."

The Coles present evidence also that number of citations is a better measure of scientific quality than productivity by showing that highly cited scientists are more likely to receive scientific awards and other forms of recognition for their work than are scientists who are highly productive but less cited. With the invention of the *Science Citation Index* it is now possible to count the number of citations to all articles in over 1,000 journals that appear in other papers published in those same journals. One can estimate in this way the usefulness of a scientific paper for the work of others. See also, Jonathan Cole and Stephen Cole, "Measuring the Quality of Sociological Research: Problems in the Use of the Science Citation Index," *The American Sociologist*, 6, No. 1 (1971): 23–29. Finally, see Chapter 4, footnote 20, *infra*.

Table 3.2   Present Religious Preference of Respondents in Our Two Studies

Present Religion	National Survey	Intensive Two-Institution Study
Protestant	44%	31%
Catholic	11	14
Jewish	17	24
None	28	31
	100% (225)	100% (369)

On the whole, then, our National Survey respondents are older, less productive in terms of quantity of publications but of higher average scientific quality as indicated by citations to their work, more likely to be Protestant, and more likely to be politically conservative. In addition as mentioned earlier, 87% of the researchers and physicians serve on their institution's P.H.S.-mandated research review committee, compared to 3% of the respondents in our second study.

For our analysis of expressed ethical standards we will rely mostly on the data from our National Survey, but we can and will supplement the analysis of two of the hypothetical proposals with responses to the same questions from our Intensive Two-Institution Study. Our analysis of reported ethical practices will, of course, come only from the second study.

Copies of our National Survey questionnaire and the interview schedule from our Two-Institution Study are reproduced in their entirety in Appendices I and II. The lengthy and detailed texts of our hypothetical research proposals appear there, and they should be read in conjunction with this immediate discussion. They are questions 41 to 46 in the National Survey questionnaire and questions 12 and 13 in the interview schedule for our second study.

ANALYSIS OF EXPRESSED ETHICAL STANDARDS

In Chapter 2 we outlined how six hypothetical research proposals involving human subjects were constructed for review by our respondents. In each proposal there were ethical dilemmas relating to how the human subjects would be treated on the consent or the risk-benefit ratio issues. All six were included in our National Survey questionnaire, and two of the six were presented to the researchers we interviewed in our second study. The replies of the respondents in both of our studies to these hypothetical proposals are used as evidence of their ethical standards as they relate to the use of human subjects in biomedical research.

Our first hypothetical research proposal in the National Survey questionnaire involved a study of the relationship between the use of hallucinogenic drugs and chromosome break. As we wrote the proposal there is no provision for the researcher's obtaining consent from the prospective student-subjects. In addition to the problem of informed consent there is the question of anonymity for the participants if they are found to be drug users. The proposal does not guarantee anonymity to the students, but it is probable that many of our respondents merely assumed that ordinary standards of privacy of communication between doctor and patient would apply here also.

Further, there is an inadequacy in the design of the study which might lead to false or inaccurate results. The means for determining drug use specified in the proposal is a urinalysis. This analysis would not detect users who have not used drugs within the length of time it takes for the drug to pass from the system. If chromosome break is related to hallucinogen use, some drug users with chromosome break would not be identified as users. Some sort of interview, questionnaire, or other means, therefore, is a needed addition in order to determine drug usage more accurately.

We intended that the "chromosome break" proposal be essentially nonproblematic on the issue of physical harm or discomfort for the subjects involved, and our respondents indeed did not find it at all physically risky. None of them mentioned this issue as a cause for concern.

In the coding of responses to all our hypothetical questions we attempted to provide a coding system that would allow all major patterns to be classified and analyzed *quantitatively*. In addition, we coded most minor patterns so that a good *qualitative* analysis could be done from computer outputs.

Let us see, then, how the respondents in our National Survey reacted to the "chromosome break" proposal. Twenty-three per cent ($N = 242$)[5] of the respondents would approve the proposal without correcting any of its deficiencies. Sixty-seven per cent of the respondents indicated that they would approve the proposal only if the revisions they specified were made in it. All of the revisions indicated as necessary by the respondents involved the problem of obtaining consent. Sixty-five per cent of those who would revise the proposal for approval ($N = 162$) indicated that the informed con-

---

[5] The sample size will vary throughout this chapter depending upon the differences in the nonresponse rates to various questions. The base for the national study is 260. When ethical standards are analyzed for respondents in our second study, the total sample size is 387. When ethical practices are discussed, using the data from the second study only, the base sample size is 321. That figure represents all respondents in the second study who were actually engaged in a research study on humans when we interviewed them.

sent of the student is required; five respondents from this group would also require parental consent. An additional 27% of those revising would require consent, but they did not specify that it be informed consent. Six of this group would require parental consent in addition. Nineteen respondents, or about 12% of the group revising, would require that anonymity be specifically assured the subjects, and two of the 19 would require parental consent in addition. The small percentage concerned about anonymity is probably the result of the fact, mentioned earlier, that most respondents assumed that ordinary standards relating to physician-patient privacy would apply. Two respondents would ask for consent to take the blood and urine samples but would not inform the students about the study.

Twelve of the group who would require revisions in the proposal ($N = 162$) pointed out the problem of determining drug users which was mentioned above. Nine respondents from the group who would revise indicated that they felt the protocol lacked detail.

Eleven respondents wanted revisions made in the proposal before they would even consider it. About 6% of the total respondents ($N = 242$) indicated that they would reject the proposal, but they also indicated that their rejection might be reversed if their objections were met. Their objections, when specified, all involved the obtaining of consent. Only one respondent indicated that he would not approve the proposal under any circumstances.

As is obvious from the data above, the problem of informed consent which we wrote into the chromosome break proposal was widely recognized by our respondents, but still 23% saw nothing wrong with doing the study without the consent of the students.

The second hypothetical proposal was intended to involve more complicated issues. In addition to a more difficult consent problem there was also an element of physical risk of an unknown amount. In this proposal the problem was to determine which of two well-accepted modes of treatment of a congenital heart defect is more effective.

The researcher in this instance was not going to inform the parents of the subjects that his choice of treatment for their children was a scientific and random one, not based on a therapeutic decision in each case. It is important to note that the hole between the ventricles, the heart defect in question, was of a size which did not unequivocally indicate either of the two modes of treatment, surgery or the "wait and see" approach. There is the risk of operative mortality if the choice is surgery when surgery may not be required and the risk of death or of a handicapped life due to the heart defect if surgery is not performed when it should be performed. In this situation, then, there is a risk involved in either choice, and the study is designed to see which therapy involves the greater statistical risk.

If the researcher in this study were careful to obtain informed consent and/or allowed parents to choose which therapy their child would receive, one or the other of his planned experimental groups might have had significantly fewer cases than necessary. In addition, some parents might have decided to go elsewhere to a surgeon who would make a decision on therapeutic grounds only, making it difficult for the researcher to obtain a sufficient number of subjects to do the study. The power of the study would, therefore, have been reduced because he could not allocate subjects to one treatment or the other in a random manner, an essential requirement of good experimental design.

In the case of this proposal only 12% ($N = 239$) of our respondents were willing to approve the proposal without revision. Fifty-five per cent would require revisions, but they would approve the proposal if the recommended revisions were made. An additional three respondents would require more information or revisions before considering the proposal at all.

Of those who would require revisions ($N = 131$), 80% would approve the study only if informed consent were obtained from the parents. Six respondents indicated that the parents should be able to choose which therapy their children would receive, while thirteen more (10%) would require informing the parents of the study in addition to allowing the parents to choose the therapy. Only a few respondents wanted different sorts of revisions and, again, nine respondents complained of insufficient detail in the write-up of the protocol. A certain percentage of complaints about lack of detail were inevitable in the approach we have taken, since very complex research proposals were being described in only a page or less of single-spaced text. Some respondents, of course, may have used such complaints to avoid making a difficult decision.

Fourteen per cent of the respondents would reject the proposal with a possible change of mind later, while 18% of the respondents would reject the proposal while indicating no possibility of approval at a later time.

Those who would reject the proposal ($N = 73$) have little consensus on their reasons. About 44% would reject at least in part because of the consent issue. Others make a choice as to which form of therapy they think is best and advocate that. Ten call the surgery in the experimental group unnecessary, while six complain that an operation which is so successful should not be withheld from the controls. Eleven respondents believe either that the data can be generated by gathering statistics from various sources already available or that the study is unimportant.

Though only 12% of our respondents would approve this study without making any revisions, only 65% ($N = 239$), on the other hand, said anything about the issue of consent. Responses to this question and to the one involving chromosome break do, on the whole, indicate that there is a fairly wide consensus among at least the majority of researchers that consent should be obtained from subjects or other responsible agents before doing any experimental procedures. There seems to be more consensus on this issue than there is on the issue of how much risk is too much in proportion to the therapeutic and other benefits, as we shall see later.

The great variety of responses to the two proposals we have analyzed so far reflects the complexity of the issues involved. Most respondents displayed careful sensitivity to the ethical issues involved, but there was still a significant percentage in both cases who saw no ethical problems of any kind with either proposal.

Our third hypothetical research proposal presents yet a third set of problems. This proposal advocates the testing in a psychiatric hospital of an antidepressant drug which appears, on the basis of early evidence, to be somewhat more effective than a widely used standard drug. It also appears, however, to cause more severe side-effects than the standard drug. In addition, the design of the study calls for the use of a placebo control group of depressed patients. A proportion of the depressed patients in the hospital are suicidal, and some of these patients would be in the control group. Written consent would be obtained from the patient-subjects or their legal guardians.

The problem, then, is to decide whether the possibility of discovering a more effective drug is worth the danger to the subjects as a result of the side-effects. In addition, there is the problem of denying treatment to the controls during the course of the study, of whom some are suicidal.

A total of 50% ($N = 242$) of our respondents indicated that they would approve the proposal as it stands. This is a much higher percentage than in the first two questions. Twenty-four per cent said that they would approve the project if it were revised. Of those who would approve the proposal if it were revised ($N = 58$), 55% said either that the controls should receive the standard drug or that the suicidal patients should be given special attention. Another 28% wanted all subjects to be carefully screened so that those susceptible to the side-effects would be excluded. Also in this group were those who insisted that any subject experiencing side-effects be dropped from the study immediately and those who wanted the experimental group limited to failures on the standard drug. In addition, 47% of those who would approve the proposal if it were revised complained of a lack of detail in the proposal as we wrote it. Only in the case of this proposal did lack of detail seem to bother a significant number of respondents.

Approximately 10% of the respondents ($N = 242$) wanted revisions made before they would consider the proposal at all. A total of 16% of the respondents would reject the proposal either completely or with some indication that their decision was not final. About 64% of those who would reject the proposal ($N = 39$) gave high risks to the subject as their reason for doing so. An additional 26% gave the withholding of treatment from the controls as their reason, but presumably they might have changed their minds if the controls were to be given the standard drug.

The responses summarized above are examples of the complex kinds of judgments that have to be made in evaluating research proposals in which human subjects will be used. The problem of withholding treatment from the controls could be taken care of by revising the research design, but then the power of the experiment might have been decreased. When respondents found that, in their judgment, the risks outweighed the benefits, some tried to devise revisions which would, if implemented, decrease the risk to the subjects. Others rejected the proposal completely under those circumstances. It should be remembered, though, that 50% of our respondents saw no ethical problems whatsoever in doing the study as we wrote it.

The second set of three hypothetical proposals was designed somewhat differently from the first set. We wanted to focus here very closely on the risks-benefits determination, and hence we made it explicit in these three proposals that the researcher would obtain consent from his subjects. Problems of consent are not totally lacking, of course, because in two of the three proposals children would be used as subjects. Obtaining an informed consent from children is an ethical problem in itself. We tried, however, to remove the issue of consent from the focus of attention.

The first two of this second set of three proposals, involving a thymectomy proposal and a study of bone metabolism, ask, essentially, what probability that an important discovery will result must be present in a study before a certain amount of risk to human subjects is justified when there will be little or no therapeutic benefit for the subjects involved. The last proposal asks what probability of a known kind of risk to the subjects is too high to approve the medically important study as proposed when, again, there will be little or no therapeutic benefit for the subjects. The last two proposals, one in slightly modified form, were the ones used in our Intensive Two-Institution Study.

The first proposal in this second set was intended as one with a potentially high payoff in terms of scientific knowledge but with very severe risks to the human subjects who might be involved. It involved thymectomizing a portion of a group of children and adolescents, who were to undergo surgery to correct heart lesions anyway, in order to see if thymectomy would increase the probability of tissue transplant survival. Each child or adolescent in the group would receive a small skin graft after the operation, and the survival of these grafts was to be compared between the thymectomized and nonthymectomized groups. The relationship between the thymus and immunological capability in children was outlined briefly in the proposal.

The phenomenon of tissue rejection in transplants has become widely known as a result of the dramatic heart and kidney transplants. Tissue transplants of many other types, such as skin grafts, are much more common though less publicized, and many physicians would ascribe great importance to solving the problem of tissue rejection.

This particular research protocol, however, involves a high degree of risk for those children and adolescents who would be thymectomized and no possible therapeutic benefit to them in return. In addition to the small added surgical risk of thymectomy during an already serious surgical procedure, there is the possibility of destruction of immune response, not only to the tissue transplants, but to various diseases to which humans have become hereditarily immune. This protocol is a rare example of a high-risk procedure coupled with no accompanying therapeutic compensation of any kind to the subjects.

It needs to be emphasized that this proposal is a very unrepresentative one. We must constantly keep in mind that only a very small proportion of clinical investigations involve high risk to the subjects with no therapeutic benefits to them in return. In our Intensive Two-Institution Study, for example, our respondents told us that out of 422 projects involving human subjects only 4 (1%) involved high risk. Two percent were reported to involve moderate risk, 8% some risk, 45% very little risk, and 44% no risk at all. Only one study involving moderate to high risk was said to have no therapeutic benefit whatsoever for the subjects. The kind of response our sample of physician-researchers gives to the thymectomy proposal is very important, therefore, precisely because the proposal is of such an extreme and rare kind.[6]

Fully 72% ($N = 232$) of the respondents in our National Survey indicated that the prospective researcher in the "thymectomy" proposal should not attempt the study no matter what the probability that the proposed investigation would establish that thymectomy considerably increases the chances of tissue transplant survival in children and adolescents. The entire distribution of responses is presented in Table 3.3.

It is comforting to note the widespread dismay among our respondents with respect to this proposal, but it is also cause for concern that as many as 28% of our respondents would approve such a high-risk study where no proportionate therapeutic benefits to the subjects are provided. Some of those respondents who would approve said, of course, that the scientific value of the study and its potential benefit to others in the future justify the risk to the present subjects, but obviously there are many researchers who do not find that reasoning compelling. The following comments by respondents are representative of this view:

---

[6] This is certainly true, even taking into account some underestimation of risk and overestimation of benefit by our respondents, to be described below.

This study can in no way benefit this patient and therefore whatever the risk, and this is unknown, it is not justified.

No therapeutic benefit for the subjects involved, who also might suffer immunological deficiencies in the future. The patients selected will undergo major surgery, risk of infection, possible bacterial endocarditis, and it's not ethical to expose them to any added risk.

Unreasonable to use patients as guinea pigs!

Patients would not benefit therapeutically. Long-term effects of thymectomy in children are unknown—could be quite deleterious.

Results probably would not justify procedures. I hope that these type experiments are not being conducted anywhere.

Table 3.3. Per Cent Willing to Approve Thymectomy Study Proposal for Each Degree of Probability of Success

1 in 10	6%
3 in 10	4
5 in 10	11
7 in 10	5
9 in 10	2
Not as proposal stands	72
	100% (232)

The fifth hypothetical proposal involved a study of bone metabolism in children suffering from a serious bone disease. It was included in our intensive interview study in exactly the same form as it was presented in the national study. The researcher in this case wanted "to determine the degree of incorporation of calcium into the bone by using radioactive calcium." He planned to use a control group of healthy children. Both groups were to be given radioactive calcium, an isotope with a long half-life, as a tracer to see how much less well the sick children absorb calcium into their bones. The radioactive calcium, however, would tend to stay in the bone and emit radioactivity in the marrow. Other studies have shown that radioactivity depresses bone marrow function and that leukemia could result. The study would have no immediate therapeutic benefit for either the experimental or control group, but the sick children might eventually benefit by the findings. As mentioned above, the researcher planned to get the informed consent of the parents of the children involved.

It was our intention in writing this proposal to make the risks to the subjects substantial but somewhat less than those in the thymectomy study. It was hoped that a study of this kind would be viewed by our respondents as important, though much less detail was given in this case about the disease involved or the exact methodology.

Our respondents in the National Survey seemed to agree with us that this hypothetical proposal to study bone metabolism was less risky than the thymectomy. About 54% of our respondents ($N = 230$) felt that the researcher should not attempt the investigation no matter what the probability that an important medical discovery would result. This compares with 72% for the thymectomy proposal. Table 3.4 gives the remainder of the distribution.

Table 3.4. Per Cent on National Survey Willing to Approve Bone Metabolism Study Proposal for Each Degree of Probability of Success

1 in 10	14%
3 in 10	4
5 in 10	13
7 in 10	8
9 in 10	7
Not as proposal stands	54
	100% (230)

The vast majority of those respondents who indicated their complete disapproval of the proposal gave as their reason that radioactive calcium should not be given to children, especially the normal controls, because of the risks of leukemia involved. The following comments are representative of this group:

Radioactive calcium should not be given to normal children. Risks are understated, underestimated, and undetermined.

Healthy volunteers should not be exposed to *any* risk, no matter how small. In my experience sooner or later "controls" come along best by careful analysis of patients who have received the drug or radionuclide or whatever for some other reason. I would never use "normal" controls.

No benefit for the subjects involved, with "only very slight" (that is enough) risk for them. I hate to be personal about it, but it seems to me that I will not allow my own children to be used as controls, and other children are as precious to their parents as mine are to me. Therefore I would not approve the proposal.

In our Intensive Two-Institution Study the response to this question was almost identical to that in the National Survey. Again, 54% of the interviewees in our second study would not approve of the bone metabolism proposal no matter what the probability of success. Fully 62% of our interviewees said in their comments that they were responding conservatively because the risks were high in relation to the benefits. Fourteen per cent of the interviewees in our second study would approve the bone metabolism study even if the chances of success were only 1 in 10, again exactly the same as the national study. Here again, then, a significant number of biomedical researchers in our studies would approve of research with potentially significant risks to the human subjects involved where no immediate benefit to them was anticipated.

Our last proposal involved a less risky procedure than the previous two proposals, and the question was changed a bit. The question, as it appeared in our National Survey questionnaire, outlined a proposal to study pulmonary function in adults under anesthesia for routine hernia repair. To obtain the data on pulmonary function the subjects would have to remain under anesthesia for an additional half hour, and hence the chance of postoperative complications such as atelectasis and pneumonia might increase. The researcher planned to obtain informed consent from each subject.

Instead of varying the probability of discovery, as in the previous two questions, we varied the probability that atelectasis and/or pneumonia might occur. In this case, then, respondents were asked to pick the highest probability (of postoperative complications) that they would consider acceptable for their approval of the proposed investigation.

In this case only 29% of our respondents would not approve the study no matter what the probability that an increase in the postoperative complications would result. This compares with 54% and 72% for the previous two proposals. An additional 42%, however, would approve the study only if there was virtually no chance of an increase in the number of postoperative complications. Many of these said that in their hospitals the chance of complications would be virtually zero if the study were done there. The remainder of the respondents spread over the other four alternatives with a smaller proportion choosing each successively more risky alternative.

Two dominant patterns of objections to the pulmonary function study were clear. One group felt that the data could be obtained without additional risk to the patient-subjects if it were done during a longer surgical procedure. In this way the subjects would not be kept under anesthesia solely for the purpose of gathering data for the study. Another group felt that there was an added risk to the subjects that was not balanced by any short-term or potential long-term benefit to them. Hence, the study should not be done.

In our Intensive Two-Institution Study the same proposal was presented with two changes. Whereas in the version for our National Survey it was stated that the researcher planned to obtain the consent of the subjects before they participated in the study, no mention of consent was made in the version for our interview study. Since we used only two proposals in this study, not six as in the other, and since we had no question specifically emphasizing consent in the second study, we needed to include this ethical problem in one of our two proposals. We wanted, in short, to see if our interviewees would notice the omission of any provision for consent. If our interviewee had completed his answer to the question without bringing in the issue of consent, we specifically asked if he thought consent necessary in a study such as that.

The second difference in the versions of the pulmonary function proposal for the two studies was in the answer format. Whereas in the National Survey questionnaire respondents were asked to choose the highest amount of risk to subjects acceptable to them, in the interview study they were just asked to approve the study as it stood, revise it in some way or reject it. They were asked their reasons if they chose to revise or reject it.

In our interview study 15% ($N = 370$) of the respondents would completely reject the proposal, mostly because they felt that the risks outweighed the benefits to the subjects involved. Seven per cent would reject the study, but would reconsider their decision if the revisions they listed were carried out. An additional 66% would require revisions in the proposal before they would approve it, while 12% of our respondents would approve the proposal as it stood. Looking at another dimension, 24% of our respondents pointed out, without a probe from us, that the researcher in our hypothetical pulmonary function study was not planning to obtain consent from his subjects. Forty-one per cent more of the respondents said that they would require the researcher to obtain consent, but they said that only after we pointed out the issue to them and asked their opinion. In 19% of the cases we failed to probe for the consent issue when it was not brought out by the respondent, but this was largely because we decided to probe in all of our interviews only after pooling our experiences as interviewers in the community and teaching hospital. In 16% of the cases our respondent specifically indicated that he would not require the researcher to obtain the consent of the subjects.

So far we have examined responses to our hypothetical proposals taking each question separately. What can we say about patterns of strictness or permissiveness in the responses we obtained? As we have said we are interested primarily in the standards our respondents express with regard to two crucial ethical issues in biomedical research on humans: the issue of voluntary informed consent and the issue of the proper ratio of risks and benefits. In our National Survey, three hypothetical proposals dealt only with the issue of risks versus benefits: the thymectomy proposal, the bone metabolism proposal, and the pulmonary function proposal. Our respondents saw the thymectomy proposal as least justifiable (72% would not approve it under any circumstances), then the bone metabolism proposal (54% would not approve it under any circumstances). Most justifiable in the eyes of our respondents was the pulmonary function proposal, with only 29% saying that they would not approve it under any circumstances.

How consistent are our respondents' judgments with regard to these questions? Only 10% of the physicians and researchers in our National Survey ($N = 260$) who answered all three questions ($N = 231$) viewed the thymectomy study as being more justifiable than the bone metabolism proposal. Seventeen per cent saw the thymectomy as more justifiable than the pulmonary function study, and 21% saw the bone metabolism study as more justifiable than the study of pulmonary function. While our respondents were not perfectly consistent, they were reasonably so. Seventeen per cent would not approve any of the three proposals, while 22% would reject none of the three. Or, according to a composite "permissiveness index" based on these three questions (see Chapter 4, footnote 22), 39% of the researchers and physicians ($N = 224$) are classified as ethically "strict" regarding the risk-benefits issue; the rest were permissive to a lesser or a greater degree.

Of the three other hypothetical proposals in our National Survey only one, the chromosome break study in a college student health center, deals exclusively with the issue of informed consent. Twenty-three per cent of the physicians and researchers who answered this question ($N = 242$) said that they would approve it as it stands, that is, the researcher who proposed the study should *not* be required to obtain consent from the students he planned to use as subjects in the study.

In our Two-Institution Study 21% ($N = 365$) would approve of the bone metabolism study if the chances of success were only 3 in 10 or less, while 16% would allow the pulmonary function study to be done without requiring the researcher to obtain informed consent from his subjects and another 41% required consent, but only after an interviewer probe.

In summary, it would appear from our analysis of responses to the hypothetical proposals in our two studies that a majority of biomedical researchers and associated physicians have ethical standards which are at least fairly strict with respect to the issue of consent. And with regard to the risk-benefits issue a majority seem to have at least moderately strict standards. However, a significant minority with respect to each issue seem to have standards that would permit them to approve of some studies which are ethically questionable to greater or lesser majorities of their peers —standards that can be called "permissive."

ANALYSIS OF ETHICAL PRACTICES

Let us look now at the reported ethical practices of the biomedical researchers we interviewed in our second study. We asked each interviewee the following question:

> For each (of your) project(s) in which humans are involved as subjects: Assuming that "risk" is defined as danger to the subject above and beyond that to which he is already exposed as a patient or as a normal, healthy person, how much risk is involved for the subjects?

We told our respondents that studies involving any risk at all, that is, approximately that which is associated with a venipuncture, should be placed in the "very little risk" category. When more than one respondent collaborated in the same study, we averaged their estimates of risk, benefits, and significance for medical knowledge in the belief that an average would be less susceptible to the effects of bias on the part of a minority of the collaborators in a study. In some cases, then, data on the characteristics of a study were provided by only one person, while in others as many as seven or eight estimates were averaged. Estimates of risk were obtained for 422 of our 424 studies, and the distribution is given in Table 3.5.

Table 3.5. Percentage of Studies According to Reported Amount of Risk for Subjects

A large amount of risk	1%
A moderate amount of risk	2
Some risk	8
Very little risk	45
No risk	44
	100% (422)

It is quite clear from the distribution in the table that very little research judged to be of significant risk by the researchers is being done in our two institutions. Only 11% of the studies are said to involve more than just "very little" risk for the subjects involved. Let us look, then, at how much therapeutic benefit our respondents anticipate for the present subjects and for patients in the future. We asked each respondent the following question:

> For each project in which humans are involved: If successful, do you feel for those subjects who are at risk that the research will provide any long- or short-term therapeutic benefits? Once again, if the project is successful, how about therapeutic benefits for others?

The estimates of benefit for each study were averaged in the same way as risk was averaged when more than one collaborator was interviewed. We obtained the distributions given in Table 3.6.[7] Our respondents report that

---

[7] The sample size in the table differs so much mainly because, for the first part of the interviewing, we asked respondents for anticipated present benefits only if some subjects were at risk. If the study involved no risk, we did not ask for the benefit. This was corrected as soon as it became apparent how important it was to have the data for all studies.

Table 3.6. Percentage of Studies According to Anticipated Amount of
Therapeutic Benefit

	Present Subjects	Patients in the Future
Great benefit	39%	51%
Some benefit	30	42
Minor benefit	14	5
Little or none	17	2
	100% (377)	100% (411)

most of their research (69%) is intended to involve at least some benefit for
the present subjects, while in 93% of the studies at least some benefit is intended as a goal for future patients. Clearly a large number of studies are
being done where the efforts of present subjects serve others in the future
to a greater extent than their efforts serve themselves. This obviously raises
important policy questions for biomedical researchers using human subjects.
For example, do researchers have the ethical obligation to tell subjects that
they are not likely to get help, or at least, not immediately? Respondents
were also asked:

> In your estimation, how significant for the advancement of medical
> knowledge is each of your projects?

Their responses are shown in Table 3.7.

Table 3.7. Percentage of Studies According to Anticipated Significance for
Medical Knowledge

Outstanding contribution	9%
Highly significant contribution	34
Greater than average contribution	24
Modest but important contribution, or, It will contribute something	33
	100% (424)

Our respondents indicate that 67% of their studies will, if successful,
involve at least a greater than average contribution to medical knowledge.
When benefits to present subjects and significance for medical knowledge
are cross-tabulated, 18% ($N = 377$) of the studies are found to have either
"great" or "some" therapeutic benefit and only modest scientific significance
(the lowest category of significance). Clearly, then, a fair number of very

practical studies are undertaken whose purpose is the relief of patient suffering in the present even though no earthshaking scientific ideas are involved.

What we have reported so far does not seem to indicate any serious problems of ethics for the research projects on which we gathered data. Let us, however, now cross-tabulate the estimated risks of our studies with their estimated benefits for the subjects involved (see Table 3.8). Both vari-

Table 3.8. Joint Distribution of Reported Risk and Anticipated Therapeutic Benefit for Subjects in Studies

Therapeutic Benefit for Subjects	No Risk	Very Little Risk	Some, Moderate, or Large Risk
Minor, little or none	11% (44)	14% (56)	2% (7)
Some	14% (56)	12% (49)	2% (10)
Great	10% (39)	19% (78)	7% (29)
Not asked	9% (36)		100% (404)

ables have been trichotomized for this table by combining the cells with the fewest cases.

We can consider the studies falling below or along the diagonal in Table 3.8 as having risk for subjects more or less counterbalanced by intended therapeutic benefit for the subjects,[8] while those studies falling above the diagonal can be classified as less favorable for subjects. In other words, by this method we construct an index in which studies falling into the "less favorable" cells, when compared with other studies in our sample, involve risk for subjects relatively high in proportion to the amount of possible therapeutic benefit for them. When this Risks-Benefits Ratio for Subjects is actually put together in this way, 18%, or 73 of the 404 studies used in our analysis are classified as "less favorable."

It should be noted that, in order to generate enough cases for the "less favorable" category of this Risks-Benefits Ratio for Subjects, we have collapsed the original categories in the risk and subject-benefit scales in our interview questions and made the following assumption: that "no risk" bal-

---

[8] Because of the situation discussed in footnote 7, there are 36 studies which were of no reported risk and unknown therapeutic benefit for subjects. In our analysis, these will be included in this category of studies having risk more or less counterbalanced by therapeutic benefit for subjects, since they do not involve risks that would need to be offset by benefits.

ances off *either* "little or no benefit" *or* the next highest category on the scale, "minor benefit"; "very little risk" balances off "some benefit"; and "some," "moderate," *or* "a large amount of risk" balances off "great benefit." However, we can justify this assumption on other grounds.

As we have suggested earlier, there was probably a tendency on the part of interviewees to underestimate the amount of what we described as "risk to the subject above and beyond that to which he is already exposed as a patient or as a normal healthy person." Similarly, it is likely that the amount of benefit for subjects, as well as for others and for the advancement of medical knowledge, was often overestimated by our respondents. Speculation about the social pressures upon these researcher–interviewees would lead us to expect some tendency on their part toward underestimation of risk, overestimation of benefit, or both.[9] Moreover, we can provide empirical evidence to support such reasoning. For example, a review of the full descriptions of the research projects reported in our interviews uncovers a number of studies in which not all the subjects at risk—for instance, normal control subjects—would derive the therapeutic benefit indicated by the researcher.[10] In addition, respondents were asked about the likely therapeutic benefit for subjects and for others "if the project is successful." Since, in fact, not all research projects are successful, wording the question this way tends to result in inflated estimates of therapeutic benefits. Then too, dimensions of cost to subjects other than risk (for example, discomfort, inconvenience, or loss of time) have not been considered. Finally, the important related question of whether voluntary consent was obtained from the subjects was not raised with respect to these studies. Thus, the way we have constructed our Risks-Benefits Ratio for Subjects more or less compensates for these circumstances.

Having made note of these points, let us look again at Table 3.8. It indicates, as might be expected, a tendency for studies that involve risks to the human subjects to also involve a countervailing possibility of therapeutic benefit for them. For, of the 229 studies in the table reported to entail risks for subjects (see the "Very little risk" and the "Some, moderate, or large risk" columns), 156, or 68%, are categorized as promising counterbalancing therapeutic benefit (insofar as they fall on or below the diagonal in the table). Thus, it may be inferred that, when a study is going to involve risk,

---

[9] In addition, with respect to underestimation of risk, we have not been able directly to take into account the degree of technical skill of the person(s) who actually performed the procedures in an investigation. How often, for example, has the amount of risk reported by respondents been that generally estimated for a given procedure *in the hands of an expert* when, in fact, it was *a novice* who performed it? On this issue, see M. H. Pappworth, *Human Guinea Pigs* (London: Routledge & Kegan Paul, 1967), p. 21.

[10] More specific details will be found in the six case studies described in Chapter 8.

the researchers in our sample usually try to make sure that it also involves a proportionate chance of benefit for the subjects.

That there should be among these biomedical researchers such common concern for provision of proportionate therapeutic benefit to the human subjects of their studies is not surprising considering that most of them are physicians and that most also work in environments governed directly by norms of the medical profession. Indeed, in the questionnaires and interviews of respondents from our National Survey and our Intensive Two-Institution Study we find suggestion of the acceptance by many of a norm that the risk of a study to subjects should not exceed the therapeutic benefit they may receive in return, *regardless* of how important the study may be for the advancement of medical science or for other patients in the future. However, the norm seems clearest with respect to studies in which there is serious risk for subjects, when there is no realistic hope of therapeutic benefit for them and when the subjects at risk include children or others who are incapable of voluntary consent. This is indicated in the National Survey in the replies of respondents who are researchers or physicians, and most of whom are also members of their institution's review committee, to our "thymectomy" proposal. This proposed study has potential for a very important increase in medical knowledge and for great therapeutic benefit to transplant patients, but would involve child and adolescent subjects in high risk with no anticipated therapeutic benefit for them in return. Fully 72% of those respondents who are researchers or physicians ($N = 232$) reject the proposal.

When, on the other hand, the subjects are voluntarily consenting adults, the risk involved is slight, and the investigation would lead to important new medical knowledge, many find a study justifiable even though it will result in little or no therapeutic benefit for the subjects involved in it. Thus, only 29% of the respondents in our National Survey who were researchers or physicians reject our "pulmonary function" proposal, which is a study of this type. Forty-two per cent of them approve if there is virtually no chance that an increase in atelectasis or pneumonia would result, that is, essentially, if there is "very little risk" to the subjects. The other 29% give responses spread over the other four alternatives, with a smaller proportion choosing each successively more risky alternative.

Having considered biomedical researchers in their role of "physician" with its emphasis on the value of therapeutic benefit for those in one's care, this finding now leads us to recall their role of "medical scientist" with its emphasis on the value of the advancement of medical knowledge and associated benefit for mankind. It seems that the lower the risk to subjects involved in a study, the more likely it is that researchers will consider scientific significance or anticipated benefit for others to be justifications more or less equal in weight to anticipated therapeutic benefit for the subjects at risk. The various authors and codes on the subject, although somewhat ambiguous, also seem to allow for scientific and general humanitarian benefits, other than therapeutic benefit for present subjects, as acceptable counterbalances to risk to subjects, especially when the risk is not great and the subjects are not children or others incapable of voluntary consent.[11]

Forty-four per cent of the studies ($N = 404$) which we use in the analysis of our Intensive Two-Institution Study were reported by the interviewees to involve "no risk," and 45% to involve "very little risk," or "approximately the amount of risk associated with a venipuncture." Because of this, even after recalling the likelihood of some underestimation of risk by the interviewees, it seems important to supplement our Risks-Benefits Ratio for Subjects with an index that contrasts the risk with *all possible* benefits, which we call our Risks–All Benefits Ratio. This supplementary index insures more complete and accurate conclusions about studies and the researchers doing them because it takes into account, simultaneously for each study, not only risk in proportion to therapeutic benefit for subjects, but also the anticipated therapeutic benefit for others in the future as well as benefit for medical science.

This supplementary index was constructed in a systematic manner similar to that used to construct the Risks–Benefits Ratio for Subjects, that is, on the basis of cross-tabulation of the variables involved. However, instead of cross-tabulation of only two variables (Table 3.8), all four variables just mentioned are involved. The category we call "least favorable" includes only those studies classified according to our first index as "less favorable"—that is, those involving risk relatively high in proportion to anticipated therapeutic benefit for subjects—*and at the same time* having relatively little counterbalancing therapeutic benefit for others and benefit for medical science.[12]

---

[11] See, for example, the principles of the Nuremberg and later codes.

[12] Not all cells of the four-variable table actually contain cases. Among the cells which do, we have constructed the "least favorable" category from the following: "*Very little risk*" (our intermediate category of risk) and "*minor, little, or no therapeutic benefit for subjects*" with "minor, little, or no therapeutic benefit for others" and "modest or some scientific significance" (8 studies); with "some therapeutic benefit for others" and "modest or some scientific significance" (11 studies); with "minor, little, or no therapeutic benefit for others" and "greater than average scientific significance" (4 studies). "*Some, moderate, or large risk*" and "*minor, little, or no therapeutic benefit for subjects*" with "some therapeutic benefit for others" and "modest or some scientific significance" (2 studies); with "minor, little, or no therapeutic benefit for others" and "greater than average scientific significance" (1 study); with "some therapeutic benefit for others" and "greater than average scientific significance" (1 study); with "some therapeutic benefit for others" and "high or outstanding scientific significance" (3 studies. These 3 studies have been included in the "least favorable" category, even though they were alleged

In other words, by this measure, 42 (58%) of the 73 studies "less favorable" for subjects are found to offer relatively compensating benefits for others or for science or for both. The remaining 31 studies, without these compensating factors—constituting 8% of all 404 studies in our analysis—thus become the "least favorable."

We hesitate to say that either the "less favorable" studies or those designated as "least favorable" are *necessarily* unethical or ethically deficient. On the other hand, neither do we claim that all the other studies are necessarily ethical. In most cases we have neither the medical expertise nor the evidence necessary to make such judgments. However, regarding the studies classified as "less favorable" and those classified as "least favorable," we do claim that, among all the clinical investigations from our Intensive Two-Institution Study, they were reported to involve the least justifiable proportion between risk and benefits—considering on the one hand, risk and only therapeutic benefits for subjects, and on the other hand, risk and benefit for subjects, for others, and for science. In other words, the studies included in these two categories are studies in which risk *at least* tends toward being in excess of benefit(s). Examples of studies that involve risks which more clearly outweigh benefits or practices which obviously are unethical will be found in Chapter 8.

In our analysis of the reported ethical practices of biomedical researchers in the following chapters we shall see the operation of social structural and cultural determinants of differential involvement in these kinds of studies most sharply and clearly—that is, involving findings with larger percentage differences based on a larger number of cases in the "less favorable" category—when we use the Risks-Benefits Ratio for Subjects. When we use the Risks–All Benefits Ratio, percentage differences associated with determinants will be found to be smaller (and based on a smaller N in the "least favorable" category), but nonetheless supportive of the first set of findings. Finally, we shall demonstrate the influence of these same determinants in some of the six case studies, including several "least justifiable" ones, discussed in Chapter 8. In other words, our argument regarding the determinants of researchers' ethical practices involves patterns that tend to hold up in analysis of decreasingly justifiable studies.

Now that we have shown how many *studies* fall into the "less favorable" and "least favorable" types, let us see how many researchers are involved in each type of study. Researchers were classified according to whether any of

to be of high scientific import, in line with the views of many researchers and physicians, discussed above, who object to research high in risk and lacking in therapeutic benefit for the human subject, regardless of its scientific significance). "*Some, moderate, or large risk*" and "*some therapeutic benefit for subjects*" with "some therapeutic benefit for others" and "modest or some scientific significance" (1 study).

their studies were either "less favorable" or "least favorable." Since most of the studies on which we gathered data were collaborative (83%), a higher percentage of researchers is involved in "less favorable" and "least favorable" studies than the percentage of studies which fall into those categories. Twenty-six per cent of the researchers interviewed were involved in at least one "less favorable" study, and 11% were involved in at least one of the "least favorable" studies. On the basis of these data it would seem that, while the large majority of our samples of biomedical researchers seems to hold and live up to high ethical standards, a significant minority may not.

One final and very important point in this discussion of the construction and meaning of our two Risks-Benefits Ratios needs to be emphasized. In constructing these ratios, which indicate the clinical research practices of respondents, as well as in constructing the earlier discussed "permissiveness index," which indicates respondents' expressed ethical standards, the studies or respondents in our two samples were defined as being *more or less* "favorable," as being *more or less* "strict" or "permissive," *in comparison to one another, not simply by reference to some absolute ethical standards.* No such standards exist. However, insofar as we do have reference to outside standards as a basis for classification, we have tried to use norms and principles found in or related to the biomedical research community itself and to the values of the society. We have not postulated arbitrary personal ethical positions as the relevant standards. In short, we have taken as references the norms which are in fact widespread among clinical investigators and among the authors of ethical codes relating to clinical research. Of course, there is no absolute or complete consensus on these ethical norms and issues, but the consensus is large enough so that it seems possible to speak of a genuine Durkheimian "moral community."

Before discussing the involvement of different classes of patients in studies with differing amounts and balances of risks and benefits, let us note further interesting relationships among the variables involved in the Risks–All Benefits Ratio. We have spoken of a widespread expectation among researchers and in the literature and ethical codes that risk for subjects should be counterbalanced, first, by benefit for subjects, but that if such benefit for the subjects is lacking, there should at least be anticipation of compensating benefits to others or to medical science. We have just presented evidence that a majority of the studies we have classified as "less favorable," that is, involving risk relatively high in proportion to therapeutic benefit for subjects, do offer compensating promise of benefit to others or to medical knowledge.

However, contrary to what some biomedical research ideologies assert, Table 3.9 shows that studies which, according to our scale, have relatively high risks in proportion to benefit for subjects *less frequently* promise great

Table 3.9. Risks-Benefits Ratio for Subjects by Anticipated Great Therapeutic Benefit for Others and by Anticipated "High" Significance of Study for Medical Knowledge

	Risk-Benefits Ratio for Subjects	
	Less Favorable	More Favorable
Great therapeutic benefit for others	19% (73)	59% (330)
"High" significance for medical knowledge	32% (73)	47% (331)

therapeutic benefit for others or "high" scientific significance[13] than do studies more favorable for subjects. In short, though the "less favorable" studies offer compensations, they are *not* more valuable for future subjects or medical science than more favorable studies.

If, in addition, significance for medical knowledge and anticipated benefit for others in the future are combined into an index to see whether studies with relatively high risk in proportion to therapeutic benefits for subjects, in comparison to those more favorable for subjects, tend also to be less often "high"[14] on both of the other two possible benefits taken simultaneously, the general finding remains (see Table 3.10).

Our data, then, provide evidence which seems to indicate that studies with less favorable Risks-Benefits Ratios for Subjects tend not to be counterbalanced by high benefits to others or to science as often as studies more favorable to subjects. This finding is surprising and noteworthy in view of the expectations of the profession. Let us now examine what kinds of patients are involved in "less" and "least favorable" studies.

It has been suggested to us by some researchers that not all social categories of people are equally likely to be asked to participate (or merely used) in studies where the risks exceed the benefits. We were told that patients who are less capable of asserting their own rights and protecting their own welfare, such as ward and clinic patients, are more often utilized as subjects in the less attractive studies. As a result we asked our respondents what proportion of their research subjects in each of their studies were private or semi-private patients as opposed to ward or clinic patients. When more than one collaborator was interviewed we averaged their estimates as before.

---

[13] "High" scientific significance combines "highly significant contribution" and "outstanding contribution."

[14] "High" on other benefits taken simultaneously combines "great therapeutic benefit for others" with "high scientific significance" (as previously defined).

Table 3.10.   Risks-Benefits Ratio for Subjects by "High" on Other Benefits
Taken Simultaneously

	Risks-Benefits Ratio for Subjects	
	Less Favorable	More Favorable
"High" on other benefits taken simultaneously	12% (73)	39% (330)

In 29% of the studies ($N = 352$) the majority of the subjects were private patients. In 36% of the studies the subjects were one-half to three-fourths ward and clinic patients, while in 36% of the studies the subjects were more than three-fourths ward and clinic patients. We shall assume that studies predominantly involving oı.e or the other type of patient will not be different on the average in the number of subjects utilized.

A completely accurate breakdown of the patient populations in our two institutions into the proportion of private and semi-private patients versus ward and clinic patients is impossible using the public information available because neither institution distinguishes in its annual report among the categories listed above as far as its out-patient department is concerned. One would think that the majority of out-patients would be clinic patients but, at least in University Hospital and Research Center, there is quite a large volume of private out-patients. For in-patients, both institutions average 56% private or semi-private and 44% ward patients.

We would need such an accurate breakdown of the proportion of ward and clinic patients in the total patient populations of our two hospitals before we could say that ward and clinic patients are more or less likely to be utilized as subjects, but that question is less important than seeing what types of studies they are involved in when they do become subjects. Tables 3.11 through 3.15 tell a tale that poses questions for biomedical research policy.

In Table 3.11, we see that studies involving at least some risk are more

Table 3.11.   Type of Patients Involved as Subjects by Reported Risk

Proportion Ward or Clinic Patients	No Risk	Very Little Risk	Some, Moderate, or Large Risk	
0– 49%	25%	29%	42%	
50– 75%	42	34	17	
76–100%	33	37	42	
	100% (145)	100% (166)	101% (41)	(367)

likely than studies of lesser risk to involve a preponderance of either private patients or ward and clinic patients, and least likely to have a more even patient breakdown.

In Table 3.12, we see that studies involving great therapeutic benefit for the subjects are more likely than those of lesser benefit to be done using subjects the majority of whom are private patients, whereas studies with minor or no benefit for subjects are most likely to involve mostly ward or clinic patients. Our data reveal that the situation is very similar when type of patients involved as subjects by anticipated therapeutic benefits for others is considered. The same is true when we look at type of patients involved as subjects by anticipated scientific significance of study (Table 3.13).

Table 3.12. Type of Patients Involved as Subjects by Anticipated Therapeutic Benefits for Subjects

Proportion Ward or Clinic Patients	Minor, Little, or None	Some	Great	
0– 49%	18%	28%	36%	
50– 75%	36	34	34	
76–100%	46	38	30	
	100% (97)	100% (102)	100% (133)	(337)

Table 3.13. Type of Patients Involved as Subjects by Anticipated Scientific Significance of Study

Proportion Ward or Clinic Patients	Some or Modest Contribution	Greater Than Average Contribution	Highly Significant or Outstanding Contribution	
0– 49%	22%	24%	36%	
50– 75%	34	35	37	
76–100%	45	41	27	
	100% (107)	100% (85)	100% (160)	(352)

Table 3.14 tells the most consequential part of our story. Studies where the risks are relatively high in proportion to the therapeutic benefits for subjects, according to our scale, are almost twice as likely as more favorable studies to be done using subjects more than three-fourths of whom are ward and/or clinic patients. In addition one cannot even say, based on Table 3.15, that the efforts of ward and clinic patients, if not for their own benefit, will at least result, on the average, in some benefit to others in the future or in

Table 3.14.   Type of Patients Involved as Subjects by Risks-Benefits Ratio for Subjects

Proportion Ward or Clinic Patients	Less Favorable	More Favorable	
0– 49%	19%	31%	
50– 75%	23	38	
76–100%	58	31	
	100% (64)	100% (288)	(352)

Table 3.15.   Type of Patients Involved as Subjects by Risks–All Benefits Ratio

Proportion Ward or Clinic Patients	Least Favorable	More Favorable	
0– 49%	17%	30%	
50– 75%	24	37	
76–100%	59	34	
	100% (29)	101% (323)	(352)

significant increases in medical knowledge. For when the Risks–All Benefits Ratio is used, where risk is contrasted to anticipated therapeutic benefit for others and possible benefit to medical knowledge as well as therapeutic benefit for subjects, the "least favorable" studies are still almost twice as likely as the more favorable to be done using three-fourths or more ward or clinic patients.[15]

The use of ward and clinic patients in the ways described above raises

---

[15] The differential treatment of ward and clinic patients as against private, paying patients has recently been the subject of much controversy in the public press with regard to the "Cincinnati Case" where, it is alleged by some and denied by others, that charity cases in a public institution who were suffering from fatal cancer were subjected to whole-body radiation on an experimental basis without their informed voluntary consent. For some reports on this case, see *Science and Government Report*, Jan. 12, 1972, p. 3, and Paul Jacobs, "The Cabinet of Dr. DOD," *New York Review of Books* (March 9, 1972), pp. 32–34.

There is apparently differential treatment of financially better- and worse-off patients with regard to kidney transplants. For some evidence, see Simmons and Simmons, "Organ Transplantation: A Societal Problem," *Social Problems*, 19 (1971): p. 43. There is even, apparently, some differential treatment of dead or dying people who arrive at the Emergency Unit of "County Hospital," studied by David Sudnow, in *Passing On: Death and Dying As Social States of Affairs* (Englewood Cliffs, N.J.: Prentice-Hall, 1967), pp. 104–109. Sudnow also comments that bodies arriving at this unit are considered as automatically suitable for teaching and research purposes.

questions of policy, of course, because those are the people who are least likely to be able to understand a study in order to give a truly informed consent. They are less knowledgeable about how hospitals are organized and about what goes on in them other than just patient care. They are least likely to be able to protect themselves personally or through legal processes against a physician who would try to take advantage of them.

Our data, then, throw light on another assumption that is held by many biomedical researchers, the assumption that, in order for medical knowledge to grow, some people have to serve as subjects for risky but important research. Those people, it is assumed, should rightly be the ward and clinic patients who receive their medical care either free or at a reduced charge. In return for cheaper care they will provide the crucial ingredient for medical knowledge to grow. While the studies with the poorest Risks-Benefits Ratio for Subjects more frequently involve ward and clinic patients than more favorable studies do, a fact consistent with the assumption in question, it is not at all clear from our data that researchers intend the sacrifice these patients make to provide important scientific or other benefits, as the rest of that assumption implies. This problem of the ethics of the differential treatment of ward and clinic patients as against private patients has not been adequately faced by the biomedical research profession. There is a moral inadequacy here that cannot be blamed entirely on the established system of payment for medical care, as it sometimes is. Even within the established system, biomedical researchers might well require, at least in this respect of medical treatment, full equality for all their patients.

It seems clear, then, that the data we have presented on the ethical standards and practices of biomedical researchers whose research involves human subjects justify the concern of people both within and outside the profession of medicine over the nature of those standards and practices. In a profession such as medicine where wide autonomy is granted to practitioners based on the long experience of others with the efficacy of medical practice and the humanitarian concern of practitioners, the patterns of behavior and attitudes we are describing can only result in a lessening of trust and therefore lead to a lessening of autonomy. These are matters we shall consider further in the last chapter.

4

THE DILEMMA OF SCIENCE AND THERAPY: THE EFFECTS OF COMPETITION IN THE SCIENCE COMMUNITY

Having described the two patterns of expressed standard and behavior with regard to the use of human subjects in biomedical research, the patterns which we have called "strict" and "permissive" and which seem to represent the more conforming and more deviant responses to moral expectations in this field, we turn now to some explanation of the social sources of these different patterns. As we have said, our explanations fall into two broad classes. One, which will occupy us in later chapters, is a class that includes three different types of social control structures and processes: socialization, collaboration groups and informal networks, and formal peer group review. The other class, to which we proceed in this and the following chapters, looks to the consequences for standards and behavior of the successful or unsuccessful resolution of potentially conflicting values in certain socially structured situations. Varying social structures, we shall show, put different pressures on biomedical researchers to be strict or permissive, to conform to or deviate from established codes. It is not so much the lack of any values, as is sometimes alleged in criticism of deviant cases, or even hypocrisy about the established values and codes, that is responsible for such behavior but rather the occasional placing of one important value ahead of another equally important value as a result of specifiable social pressures.

In the case of the biomedical research community, we have come to call this problem *the dilemma of science and therapy*. Ethical biomedical research requires the successful balancing of two important values. As physician, the researcher holds the value of humane therapeutic treatment.[1] As scientist, he holds the value of scientific success through priority of discovery.[2] Very often, these two values can both be achieved fully, or in some

---

[1] For clear and strong statements of this value, see any one of the codes that have been drawn up, from the Nuremberg Code to recent ones, on the ethics of research in medicine.

[2] On the centrality of this value for science, see Robert K. Merton, "Priorities in

ethically satisfactory balance, in a given piece of research using human subjects. Our data show this clearly. Sometimes, however, emphasis on one value may make the achievement of the other difficult. For example, too great a concern for patients in general, or for some particular patients, may prevent a researcher from carrying out a piece of work that might lead to an important discovery. On the contrary, as some researchers themselves have alleged, an ambitious researcher may press too hard with his "new" ideas and his quest for scientific recognition to the detriment of his human subjects.[3]

The social structure of competition and differential reward in science has a vital influence on the possibilities for success or lack of success in resolving this dilemma of science and therapy and on the consequent manifestation of conforming or deviant behavior. Men who are relative successes in this competition, we find, are more likely to follow the strict patterns of standard and behavior. Those who are relative failures are more likely to show the permissive patterns. Furthermore, men who are likely to feel that they have been fairly treated in the structure of competition and differential reward are more likely to be strict. Those whose situation leads us to infer that they may have been unfairly treated are more likely to be permissive.

There are two areas in which the social structure of competition and differential reward in science works itself out. One is the whole community of science, that international set of scientists (greatly subdivided by specialty and subspecialty, of course) who read each other's journal publications and express their evaluations of published scientific work by such tokens of respect and recognition as citations in their own later publications and the award of prestigious jobs, prizes, and medals.[4] The other area for competition is the local institution in which individual scientists actually carry on their research. Here, as we shall see in Chapter 5, other criteria of competence, besides scientific accomplishment, operate. In academic institutions, respect and recognition for success in the competition of science and other spheres are expressed by position in the hierarchy of professorial rank. In nonaca-

Scientific Discovery," *American Sociological Review*, 22 (Dec., 1957): 635–659, and "Resistance to the Systematic Study of Multiple Discoveries in Science," *European Journal of Sociology*, 4 (1963): 237–282; see also Warren O. Hagstrom, *The Scientific Community* (New York: Basic Books, 1965); Norman W. Storer, *The Social System of Science* (New York: Holt, Rinehart and Winston, 1966).

[3] For some evidence, see Beecher, *Experimentation on Man*, and Pappworth, *Human Guinea Pigs*.

[4] As will be seen shortly, we shall use citations as our indicator of relative evaluation, reward, and success in scientific competition. For a justification of using citations in this way, see Jonathan Cole and Stephen Cole "Measuring the Quality of Sociological Research: Problems in the Use of the Science Citation Index," *The American Sociologist*, 6, no. 1 (1971): 23–29.

demic research institutions, there is usually some other, well-recognized hierarchical structure of rank that similarly expresses differential success, recognition, and reward.

In each of these two areas, relative success or failure and feelings of fairness or unfairness in the structure of competition of science seem to influence the resolution of the dilemma of science and therapy. In this chapter, we show how relative failure in the community of science as a whole seems to lead to permissive standards and behavior. In the next chapter, we shall show how feelings of unfairness about rewards at the local-institutional level also are associated with permissive behavior in the use of human subjects. We turn now to the complex data and analysis of this chapter.

Our indicators of ethical standards, we may recall, are our respondents' choices in both of our studies about whether or not to approve a set of hypothetical research proposals which we presented to them for review. Each of the proposals, constructed with the aid of an eminent biomedical researcher and extensively pre-tested, involved a valid scientific question that was to be answered by studying a group of human subjects. An ethical problem or dilemma pertaining to one or another of the issues of informed consent or the risk-benefit ratio was involved in each proposal, and our respondents were asked about the conditions under which they would approve of the study, if at all. In our National Survey of the population of institutions in which biomedical research on humans is done, the person who responded for his institution was asked to evaluate six of these hypothetical proposals. In our second study, in which two biomedical research institutions were studied intensively, our interviewees were asked to evaluate two of the six proposals that were included in our National Survey.

In our second study, it will be remembered, we also gathered data on the kinds of human studies in which our respondents were then actually engaged. Most important among the questions we asked were these four: (1) the probable amount of risk of some injury for the subjects involved in the studies; (2) the amount of therapeutic benefit the subjects could expect *if the study were successful;* (3) the anticipated therapeutic benefit to future patients *if the study were successful;* and (4) the estimated scientific significance of the study *if it were successful.* These four questions were intended as measures of the risks and possible benefits of the studies on which we obtained information. The distributions of studies falling into different categories of risk and benefit and the construction of two risks-benefits ratios were described in the last chapter. Our first risks-benefits ratio, we may recall, is a measure of the ratio of risks of some injury to anticipated therapeutic benefits for the subjects of the studies, while the second takes into account scientific significance and possible future benefits to patients in general as well as present therapeutic benefits for subjects. They were called, accordingly, our Risks-Benefits Ratio for Subjects and our Risks–All Benefits Ratio.

We need to explain one technicality in our analysis. At least three different units of analysis are involved in our study. First, of course, is the *individual researcher*. His social background, the kinds of social relationships he has with his colleagues and others, and the kinds of informal groups of which he is a member are all treated as properties of the researcher. Second, as in the analysis presented in the previous chapter, there is the *research study* as a unit of analysis. Third, researchers appear as units of analysis in an artificial population once for every human study in which they are engaged, and the characteristics of the particular study and those of any other collaborators on that study, when aggregated, become contextual attributes of the researcher for that study. Researchers who are involved in more than one study are, therefore, counted once for each study, and researchers who happened not to be engaged in a research project when we interviewed them are not counted at all. The unit here is really not an individual, but an individual in relation to—that is, in his role pertaining to—one of his studies. A unit of analysis of the type just described is helpful in placing the individual more accurately in the social environment that exists in a particular study. It allows us to keep the various social contexts in which a researcher functions analytically separate and to test better their differential influence on expressed standards and actual behavior. We will call it our *"role" unit* of analysis.

A difficulty with this "role" approach is, of course, that we assume each unit to be independent when, in fact, those researchers who engage in more studies may be of specific social types. We have, however, controlled in each important table for the number of studies in which a researcher is engaged in order to see if the assumption of independence is justified in specific cases. In no instance did this result in the discovery of a spurious finding. Use of this role unit also makes our hypotheses somewhat harder to support, since persons engaged in more than one study who have the value of an independent variable which we predict is associated with engaging in less favorable studies must be engaged in more unfavorable than favorable studies if they are not to provide disconfirming as well as confirming evidence. If we are testing the hypothesis that young researchers more often engage in studies with less favorable Risks-Benefits Ratios for Subjects, for example, and a young researcher is engaged in two studies only one of which is unfavorable for the subjects, he provides one confirming case and one disconfirming case.

In addition, there is the problem that findings based on this role unit of analysis actually describe fewer individual researchers than would seem to be the case on examination of the tables. Using individuals who are presently engaged in a human study as the unit of analysis, our sample size is 312; using this new role unit, it is 651. All findings in this book were checked using the individual as a unit of analysis when the number of test cases was sufficiently large and, though the sample size becomes small in the more complicated tables, the findings are consistent. Whether or not the respondent was involved in any "less favorable" or "least favorable" studies was used as the dependent variable in these analyses. Contextual variables were, of course, not used in any of this checking because they had no meaning apart from their relationship to a particular study. That is why we are using the role unit here.

Unless specifically labeled otherwise, tables and other measures of association in this chapter that report data from our Intensive Two-Institution Study will use our "role unit" of analysis. Though we shall sometimes discuss these units as if they were individual researchers, in order to avoid the more abstract roles or "third units," the reader should keep in mind that in fact we are always referring to these role units.

With these technicalities about our several units of analysis explained, we move on to the main task of this chapter, the analysis of the effects of the pressures of competition in the community of science on ethical standards and practice. First let us review briefly the theory and research that has been done during the last twenty years on the nature and consequences of the competition and reward system in science by such sociologists of science as Robert K. Merton, Bernard Barber, Warren Hagstrom, Jonathan and Stephen Cole, and many others.[5] Repeated throughout many of these books and articles is the theme that scientific discoveries are important largely to

---

[5] Robert K. Merton, "The Matthew Effect in Science," *Science*, 159, no. 3810 (1968): 56–63; "Priorities in Scientific Discovery," *American Sociological Review*, 22 (Dec., 1957): 635–659; "Resistance to the Systematic Study of Multiple Discoveries in Science," *European Journal of Sociology*, 4 (1963); "Science and the Social Order" in *Social Theory and Social Structure* (Glencoe, Ill.: The Free Press, 1957), pp. 537–549; "Singletons and Multiples in Scientific Discovery," *Proceedings of the American Philosophical Society*, 105, no. 5 (1961): 470–486; Bernard Barber, *Science and the Social Order* (Glencoe, Ill.: The Free Press, 1952, and New York: Collier Books, 1962); "Resistance by Scientists to Scientific Discovery," *Science*, 134, no. 3479 (1961): 596–602; Jonathan Cole, "The Social Structure of Science—A Study of the Reward and Communication Systems of Modern Physics" (unpublished Ph.D. dissertation, Columbia University, 1969); Stephen Cole and Jonathan Cole, "Scientific Output and Recognition," *American Sociological Review*, 32 (June, 1967): 377–390; "Visibility and the Structural Bases of Awareness of Scientific Research," *American Sociological Review*, 33 (June, 1968): 397–413; Diana Crane, "Scientists at Major and Minor Universities: A Study of Productivity and Recognition," *American Sociological Review*, 30 (Oct., 1965): 699–714; Warren O. Hagstrom, *The Scientific Community* (New York: Basic Books, 1965); Norman W. Storer, *The Social System of Science* (New York: Holt, Rinehart and Winston, 1966); Harriet A. Zuckerman, "Nobel Laureates in Science: Patterns of Productivity, Collaboration, and Authorship," *American Sociological Review*, 32, no. 3 (1967): 391–403; Harriet A. Zuckerman, "Patterns of Name-Ordering Among Authors of Scientific Papers," *American Journal of Sociology*, 73 (Nov., 1968).

the extent that they are original contributions to the accumulated body of scientific knowledge. Hence, scientists are rewarded and accorded recognition by their peers in the measure that they have made original discoveries. To be original, as Merton above all has made us understand,[6] one must be the first to make a particular discovery.

In principle, of course, there are many scientific problems which, if solved, would constitute "original" contributions. If the number of such problems is well in excess of the number of scientists available to work on them, and if the solution to any of them were as likely to bring as much recognition to the successful scientist as the solution to any other, there would be little need for scientists to be competitive. Because of the role that scientific paradigms play in focusing the attention of scientists on a limited number of problems,[7] however, there is a scarcity of problems which have come to be defined as "important." Large increments of recognition come only to those who solve such "important" problems. This scarcity of opportunity to make original discoveries of a truly significant nature is a structural basis of competition among scientists.

As Merton has also said, this competition is nowhere more evident than in the endless series of priority quarrels that mark the history of science.[8] Merton has stated very well the basis for our emphasis on scientific competition as one essential determinant of all scientific work:

> The more thoroughly scientists ascribe an unlimited value to originality, the more they are in this sense dedicated to the advancement of knowledge, the greater is their involvement in the successful outcome of inquiry and their emotional vulnerability to failure.
>
> Against this cultural and social background, one can begin to glimpse the sources, other than idiosyncratic ones, of the misbehavior of individual scientists. The culture of science is, in this measure, pathogenic. It can lead scientists to develop extreme concern with recognition which is in turn the validation by peers of the worth of their work. . . . In this situation of stress, all manner of adaptive behaviors are called into play, some of these being far beyond the mores of science.[9]

How is it that taking advantage of human subjects can enable a researcher to obtain an advantage in the pursuit of scientific recognition? In

---

[6] Merton, "Priorities in Scientific Discovery," and "Singletons and Multiples in Scientific Discovery."

[7] On the focusing nature of paradigms, see Thomas S. Kuhn, *The Structure of Scientific Revolutions* (Chicago: University of Chicago Press, 1962), 25–27.

[8] Merton, "Priorities in Scientific Discovery."

[9] *Ibid.*, p. 659. Merton is, of course, only concerned here with the values internal to science, such as originality, communality, etc. He is not concerned, as we are, with the relations between these scientific values and other values, such as that of humane therapeutic treatment.

the extreme, of course, the answer is obvious. The Nazis treated humans like animals and were able to obtain data first hand that ethical researchers would have had to infer much less directly from much more complicated and sophisticated research procedures. In a less extreme case the answer is somewhat less obvious, but the following example can illustrate at least one way in which, in the competitive race for recognition, an advantage might accrue to the less scrupulous.

The use of normal controls to obtain baseline measurements for some experimental procedure generally affords the researcher the most accurate way of, say, describing the parameters of some disease state. Some procedures for obtaining measurements of normal bodily functioning do, of course, involve risk (i.e., biopsies, catheterizations). In the past, before peer review was mandated, that researcher who could bring himself to obtain data that were only obtainable using a risky procedure on normal controls which he could then compare to data from his ill subjects had an advantage in learning about the pathology of the disease he was studying. He could check the correctness of his hypothesis more quickly and more accurately. He did not need to develop subtle and less clear-cut research designs that could lead to obtaining data only in return for some possible therapeutic benefit to his subjects. In short, there were ways in which it was "rational," for the pursuit of scientific recognition, to take advantage of human subjects.

The data we have presented in Chapter 3 show, of course, that at least in the two institutions we have studied only a minority of biomedical researchers whose research involves human subjects can be said by our measures to take advantage of their subjects to any degree. It is clear that in the large majority of cases biomedical researchers can successfully balance their two central values. However, if individually felt competitive pressures to produce original discoveries can, in even a minority of cases, lead to a willingness to take advantage of human subjects, so that the research can proceed more swiftly to a solution, we must look for situations in which these pressures may be particularly acute for the types of researchers who constitute this minority. We must look more closely at actual competition in biomedical science in general and in our group of researchers.

First, how competitive is the social system of biomedical science? Warren Hagstrom[10] has used the proportion of scientists who have ever experienced anticipation of their work[11] as a measure of the amount of competition. Sixty-four per cent of Hagstrom's molecular biologists, the field on which he has data which are closest to biomedical science, reported that they had been anticipated at least once in their careers. In our studies the figures were

---

[10] *The Scientific Community* (New York: Basic Books, 1965), p. 75.

[11] For Hagstrom, a scientist may be said to have been anticipated if, after he starts work on a scientific problem another scientist publishes its solution.

of the same order of magnitude, even though Hagstrom's sample was "biased to include a disproportionate number of eminent men."[12] In our National Survey, 60% (214) of the respondents who were then presently engaged in a research project on human subjects, had been anticipated at least once. Our first study sample was weighted slightly toward higher-status men also. In our Intensive Two-Institution Study, which included many lower-status researchers because we tried to interview all researchers in the two institutions, 54% (372) of the interviewees reported that they had been anticipated at least once in their careers. Molecular biology, it must be remembered, has been a very fast-moving field ever since the discovery of DNA structure by Watson and Crick in 1953.[13] If the proportion of researchers who report having been anticipated in a field is an indicator of the amount of competition, then biomedical science must be held to be very competitive, at least as far as our respondents are concerned.

A clue as to where to look more closely for social structural bases of acute competitive pressure to achieve scientific recognition can also be found in Hagstrom's work. As he points out, the cost of experiencing an anticipation of one's work is different for established scientists and for those who are not yet established:

> Older men are more likely to have an established reputation and being anticipated on a single piece of work is not likely to affect it very much, unless the discovery is of the greatest importance. Younger men are likely to be seeking a reputation and a position, and being anticipated may negate the value of more than a year's work—a serious setback to them.[14]

To support his point, Hagstrom shows that younger scientists are in fact more likely to be concerned about the possibility of being anticipated. In his study, 29% of those receiving their Ph.D. before 1946 were concerned about being anticipated in at least one of their ongoing studies, while 65% of those receiving their degrees after 1946 were concerned.[15]

Using Hagstrom's questions, we asked the respondents in both of our studies whether they had ever been anticipated and whether they were at all concerned about this possibility in any of their present studies involving

---

[12] Hagstrom, *op. cit.*, p. 5.

[13] For an account of the discovery of DNA structure and some information about its impact on the field of molecular biology, see James D. Watson, *The Double Helix* (New York: Atheneum, 1968). The fact of competition in science and of the struggle for priority are beautifully described in this book by a working scientist. After reading Watson, the fact of scientific competition can no longer be an abstraction to any reader, scientist or nonscientist.

[14] Hagstrom, *op. cit.*, pp. 71–72.

[15] *Ibid.*, p. 71.

human subjects.[16] In our first study, 58% (90) of the respondents who were age 45 or less and who were engaged in a human study, said that they were at all concerned about the possibility of anticipation in one of their studies. Thirty-seven per cent (84) of those older than 45 said they were at all concerned. In our second study, the intensive interview study, there was about the same overall level of concern, but less spread between the two age groups. Using our third unit of analysis (since respondents were asked about their concern for each study), 55% (467) of those 45 or less were at all concerned about the possibility of anticipation, while 43% (175) of those over 45 were at all concerned. Younger respondents in both of our studies, then, were more often concerned about the possibility of being anticipated. This confirms the sociological expectation that, because younger men are in a structurally weaker position, they are more likely to fear anticipation and be aware of competition.

Age, however, our data show, is not a sufficient structural base for explaining how "strict" and "permissive" standards and practices are produced. Just being concerned about the possibility of anticipation, it turns out, is not significantly related in either of our studies to these different patterns of standard and practice. In addition, young researchers who are concerned about anticipation are not consistently different, either from young researchers who are not concerned, or from older researchers of both types in either direction on our measures of ethical standards and practices.

Fortunately, there is a good way in which we can examine the competitive pressures toward taking advantage of human subjects that result from being not yet established as a scientist. We can use a method and a typology of scientists developed by Stephen and Jonathan Cole. The Coles found it useful to examine the differential awards and rewards which accrued to physicists of four types.[17] The types, which when taken together will be called the Quality-Quantity Typology, were generated by relating the quality and quantity of scientific output of American physicists (Table 4.1). Whereas the *number of papers* published by a scientist is used to indicate

---

[16] See above where we have reported the data on the proportion who have experienced an anticipation of their work. The specific questions were as follows:

> Scientists are sometimes anticipated by others in the presentation of research findings. That is, after they have started work on a problem, another scientist publishes its solution. With respect to all of your research, clinical and otherwise, how often has this happened to you in your career? (Please exclude cases where a solution to your problem was published *before* you started your own work.) (Check only *one*.)
> For each of your studies involving human subjects, how concerned are you that you might be anticipated? (Check only *one*.)

[17] Stephen Cole and Jonathan Cole, "Scientific Output and Recognition," p. 381.

Table 4.1. Typology of Scientists According to Quality and Quantity of Published Research

	Quality	
Quantity	High	Low
High	Type I Prolific scientist	Type II Mass producer
Low	Type III Perfectionist	Type IV Silent scientist

the quality of his output in most studies which try to compare better scientists with worse ones,[18] the Coles used the *number of citations* to all of the work published by a scientist in his three most highly cited years as their indicator of the quality of the scientist.[19] The number of papers published is used by them only as a measure of the quantity of a scientist's output. They prefer citations as a measure of quality because they have found that it correlates better with scientific awards and all other expressions of recognition.[20]

Those scientists who produce many papers and are also highly cited are called "prolific scientists" by the Coles, while those who produced few papers, but were highly cited, were called "perfectionists," since even their rather low output has had a great impact on the scientific community. The terms perfectionist and prolific scientist were chosen to create the contrasting images of a patient, careful, top scientist—the perfectionist—and the perhaps less careful, less patient, but still highly competent prolific scientist. The image suggests that perfectionist scientists are less likely to publish a bad paper: they tend to publish only their best, most carefully done work. It is suggested that prolific scientists, on the other hand, may publish some bad papers in their eagerness to go into print. It is the case, as the Coles demonstrate, that the perfectionist scientist, though cited at no larger rate than the prolific scientist, is more likely to have received top awards, and perfectionists were significantly more likely to be found in the top ten departments, at least in physics. Both types, of course, were more heavily rewarded than either of the remaining two types, both of whom received few citations

---

[18] See footnote 6, *Ibid.*

[19] See Chapter 3, footnote 4.

[20] Cole and Cole, *op. cit.*, p. 385. As the Coles demonstrate in their forthcoming monograph, however, it really does not matter which of a number of different methods of aggregating citations is used. They are all highly intercorrelated and relate to other variables in the same way. See Stephen Cole and Jonathan Cole, *Social Stratification in Science* (Chicago: University of Chicago Press, forthcoming).

to their work. Those scientists who published a lot of papers, but were little cited, were called "mass producers" by the Coles, and those with few papers and few citations were called "nonproducers," or "silent scientists."

As our own data show, however, the perfectionist pays a small price. Perfectionists in our first study were more likely than any other type to have been anticipated at least once in their careers (Table 4.2). The same

Table 4.2. Per Cent Anticipated at Least Once by Quality-Quantity Typology for Respondents in National Survey

| | Quality | |
Quantity	More Than 7 Citations	0–7 Citations
More than 7 papers	Prolific scientist 82% (50)	Mass producer 69% (16)
0–7 Papers	Perfectionist 97% (29)	Silent scientist 41% (68)

table cannot be presented for our second study, because there were only 8 perfectionists among our interviewees, using the same criteria applied to respondents in our first study. The cutting points were set at 7 for both productivity and citations because the median of both distributions is close to 7 in our National Survey.

We are most interested, among these four types, in the mass producer. His high productivity is an indication that he has been working hard but that he has not been rewarded to any great extent by the scientific community in the form of citations to his work. Since having one's work form the basis for the work of others is a sign of becoming an established scientist, these researchers are clearly not yet established. In contrast to the silent scientists, who are also not yet established, however, the mass producer's continuous productivity demonstrates that he is motivated toward that end. One would expect, then, that researchers of this type would be more anxious about priority than researchers of the other types and that, in turn, they would be more concerned about the possibility of anticipation in their current research. That seems to be the case for the respondents in our first study, as Table 4.3 shows, though not for those in our second.

Let us see now if our mass producers, those researchers who are clearly not yet established but who are apparently still motivated toward that end, do tend to have permissive standards as well as a greater tendency to engage

Table 4.3. Per Cent Concerned about Anticipation by Quality-Quantity Typology for Respondents in National Survey

	Quality	
Quantity	More Than 7 Citations	0–7 Citations
More than 7 papers	Prolific scientist 60% (50)	Mass producer 79% (14)
0–7 Papers	Perfectionist 67% (21)	Silent scientist 26% (49)

in "less favorable" and "least favorable" studies according to our measures. The first hypothetical research proposal presented to our respondents for review in our first study was a proposal to examine the effects of psychoactive drug usage on chromosome break. The study was to be done in a university student health center by taking blood and urine samples from all students who visited the center without first asking for their consent. Our respondents were asked to approve or disapprove of the study exactly as presented and to explain their answer if they disapproved of the study. The data are presented in Table 4.4.

The chromosome break proposal was one in which the issue of informed consent was at the center of attention, and our mass producers were clearly more likely to approve the study as it stood without requiring, in addition, that consent be obtained from the students. Since the number of cases is small for the mass producers, our inference can only be tentative, but the consistency of this table with many others that will be presented is significant.

While we are on the issue of informed consent, we may note that the second of the two hypothetical proposals we presented in our two-institution study also involved the issue of whether or not the researcher planned to get consent from his subjects before studying them while they were under anesthesia for routine hernia repair. In fact, the researcher planned to extend anesthesia for an additional half-hour to perform the necessary tests for his study. This proposal, as discussed in the previous chapter, was an altered form of the sixth hypothetical proposal from our National Survey. As presented in our Intensive Two-Institution Study, the proposal said nothing about whether or not the researcher planned to obtain consent from the subjects before he went ahead with his study. Respondents were classified according to whether or not they noticed this absence of any provision for obtaining consent in the proposed study.

Table 4.4. Per Cent Approving Chromosome Break Proposal in National Survey by Quality-Quantity Typology

Quantity	Quality	
	More Than 7 Citations	0–7 Citations
More than 7 papers	Prolific scientist 25% (44)	Mass producer 47% (15)
0–7 Papers	Perfec- tionist 22% (27)	Silent scientist 20% (61)

In Tables 4.5 and 4.7 to 4.10, because of the paucity of perfectionists in the group of interviewees in our second study, highly cited interviewees are combined into one category, called "high quality." In addition, because no differences were observed between mass producers and the other types using our old cutting points, we have subdivided the mass producers into two categories: those with more than ten papers and one to seven citations are called "moderate mass producers," while those with more than ten papers and zero citations are called "extreme mass producers." When the mass producers were further subdivided in this way, the extreme group was clearly least likely to have noticed the lack of provision for consent in the proposed pulmonary function study. In the two hypothetical proposals which most clearly posed the issue of consent, then, mass producers were least likely to say that consent is required before a researcher has the right to use a human as a subject for an experiment.

As an illustration of processes that go into producing the relationship shown in Table 4.5, one of our interviewees outlined how the pressures to publish that he felt led him more and more toward obtaining a less voluntary and less informed consent from his subjects. Due to the length of the question response the interviewer was only able to paraphrase it, as follows:

> When he began to do his own research as a resident, he still saw things more as a physician than a researcher and was shocked at the tactics researchers used to get consent from subjects. When he became a research fellow, he was told by his senior-researcher mentor to get informed consent from subjects, and he rather scrupulously tried to do so. But he soon learned of the actual practice in this respect when he saw his senior-researcher mentor "sell" a patient on becoming a subject by "stretching the truth" about the potential benefits the patient might hope for. Also, he realized that his rewards as a researcher lay in publishing, and that his more honest, detailed, informing of patients rather frequently resulted in their refusal to be subjects so that it would

Table 4.5. Per Cent in Two-Institution Study Noticing Absence of Provision for Consent in Pulmonary Function Proposal by Quality-Quantity Typology

Quantity	Quality		
	More Than 7 Citations	0–7 Citations	Zero Citations
More than 10 papers	High quality 32% (187)	Mod. mass producer 42% (65)	Ext. mass producer 11% (28)
0–10 papers		Silent scientists 19% (294)	

take him longer to do studies (if he could get enough subjects to do them at all) and, therefore, to gain a name and advancement.

Returning again to our National Survey study, our data in that study showed that mass producers were no more and no less likely to give permissive responses to the congenital heart defect proposal or to the antidepressant drug test proposal, our second and third hypotheticals. In these two hypotheticals, the issues of consent and of risk versus benefit were both present.

The last three hypothetical proposals in our National Survey study all involved only the issue of risks versus therapeutic benefits for subjects, and so responses to these three proposals were combined into a "permissiveness index." The three proposals involved, in turn, a very risky thymectomy study to be done on children, in which no therapeutic benefit was intended for the subjects; a moderately risky bone metabolism study in which radioactive calcium was to be used as a tracer in normal and sick children, and in which little or no therapeutic benefit was intended for the subjects; and the same pulmonary function study we just analyzed, which was to involve adults as subjects. The pulmonary function study might be said by a few physicians to involve some very small benefit to the subjects, because of the likelihood that increased medical attention would be given to the patients during the study that they might not have had during a normal hernia operation, but it too had its risks. A composite "permissiveness index" based on respondents' decisions with respect to these three hypothetical proposals permits us to classify respondents as having "relatively permissive," "less permissive,"[21] or "strict" ethical standards concerning the risks-benefits issues.[22]

---

[21] See Appendix I again to see how the degrees of probability were categorized for these hypothetical proposals.

[22] This "permissiveness index" based on the replies of National Survey respondents

As in the previous two examples in which consent was the issue, when risks in relation to benefits is the issue, the mass producers in our first study were most likely to be permissive. See Table 4.6.

Table 4.6. Per Cent Relatively Permissive on Permissiveness Index by Quality-Quantity Typology in National Survey[a]

	Quality	
Quantity	More Than 7 Citations	0–7 Citations
More than 7 papers	Prolific scientist 28% (46)	Mass producer 53% (15)
0–7 Papers	Perfectionist 19% (28)	Silent scientist 30% (64)

[a] The variation in the number of cases for tables from our first study is due to variation in the nonresponse rate to the different hypothetical proposals.

The very same bone metabolism proposal, which was presented to respondents in our National Survey, and the responses to which form part of the permissiveness index just discussed, was also asked of interviewees in our Intensive Two-Institution Study. Extreme mass producers were no more and no less likely to give permissive responses to this hypothetical proposal in our second study. Because the relationship between our Quality-Quantity Typology and our indicators of expressed ethical standards is not consistent, the finding just presented is to be taken as only suggestive.

In any case, while it is important to see what factors make for higher and lower *expressed ethical standards*, it is more important for the welfare of human subjects to be able to identify factors that are related to higher and

to the last three hypothetical proposals presented in the questionnaire sent to them is constructed in the following way: Essentially, the respondents classified as "strict" regarding the risk-benefits issue are those who refused to approve the "thymectomy" and the "bone metabolism" proposals as presented, regardless of the probability of important medical discovery, and also rejected the "pulmonary function" proposal or, at least, approved it only if there was virtually no chance of an increase in postoperative complications in the subjects. The "relatively permissive" category was constructed so that it would include approximately that third of the sample who made more permissive combinations of decisions regarding the proposals than the other two-thirds majority of respondents—hence the designation, "*relatively* permissive." (For some specific percentages regarding those choosing the more permissive replies to the proposals, see Chapter 3). The remaining respondents were those who made "less permissive" combinations of replies.

lower quality *ethical practices*. The crucial test of our hypothesis that competitive pressures on biomedical researchers to make original scientific contributions lead to taking advantage of human subjects, then, is to see whether extreme mass producers in our Intensive Two-Institution Study are more likely to engage in studies where the risks are relatively high in proportion to the therapeutic benefits for the subjects (less favorable studies according to our Risks-Benefits Ratio for Subjects) and also in studies where the risks are relatively high in proportion to all benefits, that is, for subjects, for others, and for science (least favorable studies according to our Risks-All Benefits Ratio). The comparative data are presented in Table 4.7.

Table 4.7. Per Cents Engaged in Less Favorable and Least Favorable Studies by Quality-Quantity Typology

| | Quality-Quantity Typology | | | |
	High Quality	Moderate Mass Producer	Extreme Mass Producer	Silent Scientist
% Engaged in less favorable studies	20% (196)	15% (69)	39 % (28)	18% (302)
% Engaged in least favorable studies	9% (196)	7% (69)	18% (28)	6% (302)

Let us now examine what happens to the relationships in Table 4.7 for extreme mass producers who, in addition to having been productive in the past, are now engaged in a greater or lesser number of studies. Extreme mass producers who are engaged in a larger number of studies involving humans may thereby be expressing their greater motivation toward success when compared with less active extreme mass producers and other types.

First, extreme mass producers are more likely to be engaged in three or more studies involving humans than are any of the other three types. An interesting comparison can be made in Table 4.8 between the two types of mass producers. The two groups have been equally productive in the past, but the group which is less established is working hardest now.[23]

---

[23] It has not escaped our attention that in tables using the Quality-Quantity Typology the moderate mass producers often turn out to be the least permissive type. In addition to being involved with fewer studies now, they are also older, on the average, than extreme mass producers. This fact will take on importance when, below, we report that young extreme mass producers have more permissive ethical practices than young members of other types. In addition, moderate mass producers, according to other data, may have been more likely to have had socialization experiences of a type which we found

Table 4.8. Per Cent Engaged in Three or More Studies by Quality-Quantity Typology

| Unit of Analysis | Quality-Quantity Typology | | | |
	High Quality	Moderate Mass Producer	Extreme Mass Producer	Silent Scientist
Role	66% (196)	45% (69)	86% (28)	39% (301)
Individual	44% (84)	35% (34)	64% (11)	21% (177)

Table 4.9 suggests that for researchers engaged in three or more studies involving humans, extreme mass producers are the type most likely to be engaged in less favorable and least favorable studies. In fact, for those en-

Table 4.9. Per Cents Engaged in Less Favorable and Least Favorable Studies by Quality-Quantity Typology and Number of Studies

Per Cent Engaged in Less Favorable Studies

| Number of Studies | Quality-Quantity Typology | | | |
	High Quality	Moderate Mass Producers	Extreme Mass Producers	Silent Scientists
One or two	23% (66)	13% (31)	0% (4)	21% (183)
3 or more	19% (130)	16% (38)	46% (24)[a]	12% (118)

Per Cent Engaged in Least Favorable Studies

One or two	11% (66)	7% (31)	0% (4)	7% (183)
3 or more	8% (130)	8% (38)	21% (24)[b]	5% (118)

[a] + 7% when compared to Table 4.7.
[b] + 3% when compared to Table 4.7.

gaged in three or more studies, the difference between the extreme mass producers and the other types has increased when compared with the original two-variable relationship between the Quality-Quantity Typology and the risks-benefits ratios.

Thus, it is the *more active* extreme mass producers who are more likely to take advantage of human subjects in their studies. The number of studies

contributed to producing stricter ethical standards. It appears, in summary, that moderate mass producers may be a distinctive social type rather than just the type which is ordinally closest to extreme mass producers.

in which our respondents were engaged did not alter the previously reported findings with respect to the two hypothetical proposals presented in our second study. There was still no relationship between the Quality-Quantity Typology and responses to the bone metabolism proposal, and the finding that extreme mass producers were less sensitive to the issue of consent in the pulmonary function proposal was not enhanced or diminished for more active researchers.

Earlier, we noted the strong competitive pressures on younger researchers who are not yet established, as indicated by the fact that others do not cite their work. These pressures show up clearly when we compare our different quality-quantity types while controlling for age. It is our *young*[24] extreme mass producers who are most likely to be engaged in studies where the risks-benefits ratios are unfavorable for the subjects. Again, as in the case of the number of studies in which the researcher is involved, the difference between the extreme mass producers and the other types generally increased slightly when compared with the original two-variable relationship between the Quality-Quantity Typology and the risks-benefits ratios (see Table 4.10).

In summary, we have presented evidence that the pressures of having to establish oneself in a competitive scientific community seem to have the effect of making those researchers engaged in studies with human subjects who feel the pressures most acutely less sensitive to the issue of informed consent and more willing to engage in studies with less favorable risks-benefits ratios. Extreme mass producers who were engaged in three or more research studies on humans, those conforming most closely to the image embodied in the name of the type, were the ones most likely to have lower quality ethical practices. Those extreme mass producers who could be expected to feel the competition most intensely, the young ones, were also most likely to have lower quality ethical practices.

One difficulty, of course, with the way in which our analysis has proceeded so far is the continual lack of sufficient cases to insure reliable results in tables into which one or more controls have been introduced. A partial correlation analysis would seem to be the logical choice in order to circumvent this difficulty, but the effects described are almost all nonlinear. Citations, age, and number of studies do not affect the risks-benefits ratio in a linear fashion. Productivity, as we shall see, does have a linear effect, but only under certain conditions. In short, we are dealing here with interactive effects whose impact on the dependent variables in question would be masked under the assumptions of linearity in partial correlation analysis.

---

[24] Because we will need to collapse our age categories in later tables in order to introduce further controls, "young" will now be 26–39 years of age. Earlier in this chapter age was dichotomized at 45, but 39 is closer to the median.

Table 4.10. Per Cents Engaged in Less Favorable and Least Favorable Studies by Quality-Quantity Typology and Age

| | Quality-Quantity Typology | | | |
Age	High Quality	Moderate Mass Producer	Extreme Mass Producer	Silent Scientist
Per Cent Engaged in Less Favorable Studies				
26–39	35% (52)	12% (25)	44% (16) [a]	17% (196)
Over 39	15% (144)	17% (41)	33% (12)	19% (106)
Per Cent Engaged in Least Favorable Studies				
26–39	15% (52)	0% (25)	31% (16) [b]	7% (196)
Over 39	6% (144)	12% (41)	0% (12)	5% (106)

[a] + 5% when compared with percentage in Table 4.7.
[b] + 13% when compared with percentage in Table 4.7.

A way out of the difficulty does exist, however. It is possible to use the correlation coefficient to examine the relationship between one independent variable and the risks-benefits ratios for all cases within particular interactive cells in a contingency table. If our analysis so far has been correct, for researchers with zero citations increasing productivity should be related to participating in studies with less favorable risks-benefits ratios. The more, in other words, a researcher conforms to our image of an extreme mass producer the more likely he is to participate in less favorable studies. Under certain conditions, therefore, productivity should be correlated with the risks-benefits ratios.

As Table 4.11 shows, for the sample as a whole none of the variables introduced so far in this chapter is at all related to either the Risks-Benefits

Table 4.11. Productivity, Citations, Age, and Number of Studies by Risks-Benefits Ratio for Subjects and Risks–All Benefits Ratio

	Risks-Benefits Ratio for Subjects	Risks–All Benefits Ratio
Productivity	—.03	—.02
Citations	.03	.04
Age	—.06	—.03
Number of studies	.01	—.03
N = 630		

Ratio for Subjects or the Risks–All Benefits Ratio.[25] These nonrelationships are to be expected, of course, if our findings are truly in part interaction effects. Let us see how the relationships change if we look only at those researchers with zero citations. Extreme mass producers, it will be remembered, were defined as having zero citations and more than 10 papers in the last five years. Table 4.12 shows the relationships of productivity, age, and number

Table 4.12. Productivity, Age, and Number of Studies by Risks-Benefits Ratio for Subjects and Risks–All Benefits Ratio for Those with Zero Citations

	Risks-Benefits Ratio for Subjects	Risks–All Benefits Ratio
Productivity	.05	.09
Age	—.06	—.06
Number of studies	—.01	—.02
$N = 263$		

of studies with the two risks-benefits ratios for those with zero citations. These correlations are small also, but at least in the cases of productivity and age they are now in the expected direction.

With further partitioning of the data, however, our expected relationship begins to emerge. As we introduce these further controls we are beginning to examine those who more closely fit our conception of the "extreme mass producer." Table 4.13 shows the correlations of productivity and age with the risks-benefits ratios for those with zero citations who were also engaged in three or more studies on humans at the time of interview. And Table 4.14 shows the correlations for those with zero citations who are less than 40 years old. Tables 4.13 and 4.14 are analogous to Tables 4.9 and 4.10. In both we see small but noteworthy correlations between productivity and the risks-benefits ratios. However, because we have more cases to work with using this method, we can specify the relationship much further.

Table 4.15 shows the correlation between productivity and the risks-benefits ratios for those with zero citations who are less than 40 years old and engaged in three or more studies at the time of interview. Both correlations are higher than in previous tables showing that the more we isolate those who most approximate our extreme mass producers, the more likely they are to engage in studies with unfavorable risks-benefits ratios.

One final way of looking at this relationship lends even more weight to our analysis. If we also partition productivity and then examine the rela-

---

[25] The Pearson product-moment correlation coefficient is used as our measure of linear relationship throughout the subsequent analysis in this chapter.

Table 4.13. Productivity and Age by Risks-Benefits Ratio for Subjects and Risks–All Benefits Ratio for Those Engaged in Three or More Human Studies with Zero Citations

	Risks-Benefits Ratio for Subjects	Risks–All Benefits Ratio
Productivity	.15	.26
Age	—.05	.00
$N = 121$		

Table 4.14. Productivity and Number of Studies by Risks-Benefits Ratio for Subjects and Risks–All Benefits Ratio for Those Less Than Forty Years Old with Zero Citations

	Risks-Benefits Ratio for Subjects	Risks–All Benefits Ratio
Productivity	.16	.15
Number of Studies	.00	—.04
$N = 187$		

Table 4.15. Productivity by Risks-Benefits Ratio for Subjects and Risks–All Benefits Ratio for Those with Zero Citations Who Are Less Than 40 Years Old and Engaged in Three or More Human Studies

	Risks-Benefits Ratio for Subjects	Risks–All Benefits Ratio
Productivity	.28	.30
$N = 88$		

tionship between even higher productivity and the risks-benefits ratios, our largest correlation coefficients result. Table 4.16 also shows that for this group age is negatively related to the risks-benefits ratios. For those with zero citations and more than seven papers, then, it is the younger ones who are more likely to be involved in the less favorable studies.

Though the differences have been slight, the relationship between productivity and the Risks–All Benefits Ratio has tended to be larger than that between productivity and the Risks-Benefits Ratio for Subjects. That is to be expected if we are really on the right track, because the Risks–All Benefits Ratio is the stiffer test of our hypotheses.

It must be recognized here that, because of the greatly differing number of cases involved, University Hospital and Research Center, as against Com-

Table 4.16.   Productivity and Age by Risks-Benefits Ratio for Subjects and Risks–All Benefits Ratio for Those with More Than 7 Papers and Engaged in Three or More Studies at Time of Interview

	Risks-Benefits Ratio for Subjects	Risks–All Benefits Ratio
Productivity	.40	.47
Age	−.25	−.15
N = 51		

munity and Teaching Hospital, contributes most of the findings we have outlined. If we were to look only at University Hospital, in fact, the differences reported would be somewhat larger but with fewer overall cases for analysis. That, too, is as it should be because, of the two institutions, there is a much heavier emphasis on science at University Hospital and Research Center as we indicated earlier. In the interests of representativeness, however, we have decided to report findings for the two institutions combined. The findings are a little less strong, but thereby we probably come closer to representing the whole picture of biomedical research.

These slight differences between University Hospital and Research Center and Community and Teaching Hospital do not, of course, obscure our main findings. While competition among scientists for recognition and reward may have the salutary effect of increasing the overall rate of scientific advance, our findings make it clear that it has some negative consequences for other important human values, in this case the value of humane therapy. Those biomedical researchers who are failures in the social structure of scientific competition but who are still striving to achieve success in that competition are more likely than others to be those who have the permissive standards and behavior with regard to the use of human subjects in research. Our biomedical researchers, we see, are faced not only with the dilemma of science and therapy but are subject to differential pressures from the structure of scientific competition for recognition and reward. Those who succeed in this competition face pressures they can cope with while adequately resolving the dilemma through a balancing of the two values. Those who fail experience a pressure that makes them put science above therapy, thus leading to permissive and deviant standards and practices. Any attempt to reduce the amount of such deviance in biomedical research must, therefore, look to the effects of the structure of scientific competition as well as to the established values that are supposed to control researchers' behavior in this field.

In Chapter 5 we shall look at how the structure of scientific competition influences the dilemma of science and therapy in the local-institutional setting in which individual researchers actually work.

5

THE DILEMMA OF SCIENCE AND THERAPY: THE EFFECTS OF COMPETITION IN THE LOCAL INSTITUTION

In Chapter 4 we examined the effects of the structure of competition for recognition and reward in the scientific community at large on biomedical researchers' expressed standards and actual behavior in the use of human subjects. In this chapter we will show that somewhat analogous effects of the structure of competition in science exist at the local-institutional level where the individual researcher carries out his work and where the reward he seeks is organizational rank and its associated perquisites.

Sociologists of science have long asserted, but without systematic empirical evidence, that the value of *universalism* is an essential constituent in the small set of central values in science.[1] This is the value that proclaims that men should receive rewards entirely on the basis of their achievements and demonstrated merit, without reference to any of their ascribed characteristics such as race, or sex, or ethnic or family affiliation. Now Jonathan and Stephen Cole have given solid empirical support for the actual prevalence of this value in science.[2] On the basis of several studies which they have done, the Coles present systematic evidence for the proposition that, certainly in physics where most of their data come from but also inferentially for the other natural sciences, the reward system of the scientific community at large does operate in a universalistic way, that is, on the basis of the quality of scientific work published and not on the presence or absence of irrelevant individual qualities, or on occupancy of esteemed social statuses, or on mere quantity of scientific output. No other variable introduced into the analysis of their data explained a significant amount of the variance on receipt of such prestigious scientific awards as the Nobel Prize, the Fermi Award, or a

---

[1] See, for example, Robert K. Merton, "Science and The Social Order," *Philosophy of Science*, 5 (1938): 321–337; and Bernard Barber, *Science and The Social Order* (Glencoe, Ill.: The Free Press, 1952, and New York: Collier Books, 1962).

[2] In *Social Stratification in Science* (Chicago: University of Chicago Press, forthcoming).

variety of lesser awards beyond the amount explained by the number of citations to the successful and prestigious scientists' work.[3] Their data and their analysis suggest that the scientific community at large, especially already in physics, may very well approximate what Michael Young has called a "meritocracy" when it comes to the allocation of rewards for scientific achievement.[4]

Although universalistic merit is just as important in local scientific institutions, one would not expect quality of research output to be the sole basis of local-institutional rank, however, and our data show that to be the case. Other kinds of work outputs are both valued and functionally required by biomedical research organizations besides research outputs. Therapeutic and administrative skills are also needed, and some other skills researchers might have could also form the basis for achieving high local-institutional rank. For example, in the government basic research organization whose biomedical researchers Glaser studied, promotion was officially based on the following multidimensional process:

> A sample of his publications is read; prior and current supervisors are asked about him; and his qualifications are judged on: (1) the quality of work engaged in; (2) capacity to develop; (3) capability in relation to other investigators; (4) reputation in his field; (5) personal characteristics and ability to get along with others; and (6) ability in the nonscientific work associated with both his present post and his prospective position. If he passes this examination, he is recommended to the director of the organization for promotion and the director generally follows the advice of the Board.[5]

In the following pages we will describe the workings of the actual reward structures in our two local institutions. We will show what characteristics are related to the achievement of high rank. We will try also to demonstrate that researchers who are *relatively deprived* by the local reward system in that they have not been rewarded with higher rank after achieving on one or more of the criteria on which promotion is based are more likely to be involved in studies with less favorable risks-benefits ratios. We will argue that they become involved in such studies more frequently for reasons similar to those which we presented for extreme mass producers in our earlier analysis. That is, in order to increase their chances for the promotion they have not received on other grounds, they try to become more productive

---

[3] As mentioned earlier, the Coles have shown that number of citations is a valid and convenient indicator to use for measuring quality of scientific work.

[4] Michael Young, *The Rise of the Meritocracy, 1870–2033* (London: Thames and Hudson, 1958). The Coles point out some of the strains that meritocracy brings about in science, as well as its essential functions for scientific discovery.

[5] Barney G. Glaser, *Organizational Scientists: their Professional Careers* (Indianapolis: Bobbs-Merrill, 1964), pp. 5–6.

in the research area. Because, as we suggested in the last chapter, taking advantage of human subjects can sometimes enable researchers to get better data quicker, these underrewarded researchers more frequently become involved in studies with unfavorable risks-benefits ratios for the subjects.

Let us see first, then, what characteristics of researchers are related to the achievement of high rank in our two local institutions. Table 5.1 shows the zero-order correlations (Pearson) between a number of variables and local-institutional rank. The first four variables need no explanation, but the last is new to the analysis.[6] For complete clarity all will be defined:

Age: Number of years old.
Seniority: Number of years employed in the institution.
Productivity: Number of scientific papers published in past five years.
Citations: Number of citations in 1968 *Science Citation Index* to all papers published by the researcher in his three most highly cited years of work.
Consults: Number of times in month previous to interview that another physician in the institution came to the researcher being interviewed to confer informally on one of the physician's cases or therapeutic problems.[7]

Looking just at the zero-order correlations presented in Table 5.1, some expected results and some partial surprises may be observed. In bureaucratic institutions one would certainly expect to find rank correlated with age, seniority, productivity, citations and number of consults. All are indicators

---

[6] Three or four other variables than these have small but significant correlation coefficients with rank, but except in the case of religion they disappear when controls are introduced. The case of religion is very complicated, and it will be dealt with in a later paper. Exclusion of religion from this analysis in no way invalidates our analysis of the five factors we do present.

[7] The concept for which each of the above variables is an indicator seems relatively clear in all but the case of number of consults. The intent of the question which produced the responses used as the basis for this variable was merely to identify social relationships between our researchers that were based on frequent therapeutic referrals. As such, it was not intended as a reputational measure of therapeutic competence in the manner in which we will now temporarily use it. In addition, even though we asked for informal consultations that were not formally defined into institutional roles (i.e., residents must consult their superiors), it is still quite possible that in our data differential rank results in referrals as often as referrals indicate therapeutic competence which has been recognized and rewarded by the institution in the form of rank. Since physicians often receive fees when patients are referred to them by another physician or when one physician asks another for an opinion, referrals are actually a form of reward in many cases also. Because of the lack of precision in this variable, it will not be part of the analysis of the whole chapter but will be dropped after our initial discussion.

Table 5.1. Pearson Correlations of All Variables with Rank[8]

Age	.53	(582)
Seniority	.47	(582)
Productivity	.41	(582)
Citations	.36	(582)
Consults	.17	(542)[a]

[a] Number of cases is low because only physicians have therapeutic consultations and some researchers are not physicians.

of characteristics of people that we have come to accept as bases for the possession of high rank in formal organizations. Somewhat surprising, however, are the relative strengths of these relationships in our two biomedical organizations. Age and seniority correlate much more highly with rank than anything else, and productivity and rank are more related than citations and rank. This is an early indication of the extent of the differences between the local-institutional and larger scientific reward systems. Because of their functional requirements for input of other things than just scientific quality, local institutions have to acknowledge and reward other qualities as well.[9]

Before we make unwarranted conclusions, however, it is essential for us to see the degree to which each of these factors affect rank when the others are simultaneously controlled. Table 5.2 shows the partial correlations

Table 5.2. Fourth-Order Partials, Each Variable Correlated with Rank Controlling for the Other Four Variables

Age with rank	.32
Citations	.23
Productivity	.20
Consults	.17
Seniority	.13

between rank and each of its five bases with the other four variables simultaneously controlled. The coefficients above suggest that each of the five variables tested have independent effects on level of institutional rank. Note that productivity, an indicator of mere quantity of research output, is seen to have a significant independent effect on rank almost as large as that for research quality as measured by citations. Note too that age remains the most

---

[8] Correlations are computed using our "role" unit of analysis because later that unit is related to our dependent variables and not the individual as a unit. When the correlations are computed using the individual as the unit of analysis, they are almost identical.

[9] On this matter, see Glaser, *Organizational Scientists*, Chapter 2, "The Local-Cosmopolitan Scientist."

important factor in the achievement of institutional rank. While some young high-quality researchers seem to be able to obtain early rewards, so too can older, lower-quality researchers eventually achieve high rank on the basis of their performance of other functions. Some of the implications of this point will be examined in detail below.

The two institutions we selected for study, it will be remembered, differ from each other on a number of dimensions. University Hospital and Research Center is a high-quality medical school–teaching hospital complex, while Community and Teaching Hospital is a more therapeutically oriented hospital where research is emphasized to a lesser degree. These differences were evident in the comparison between the institutions we presented in Chapter 2. We should not be surprised, then, to find differences in their institutional reward structures, and there are indeed interesting differences. Table 5.3 presents the fourth-order partials of each of our five variables

Table 5.3. Fourth-Order Partials, Each Variable Correlated with Rank Controlling for the Other Four Variables by Research Institution

	University Hospital and Research Center	Community and Teaching Hospital
Age with rank	.32	.29
Citations	.28	.02
Productivity	.11	.24
Consults	.17	.15
Seniority	.14	.23

with institutional rank, controlling for the other four, separately for our two institutions. The correlations between age and rank and consults and rank are about the same for the two institutions. At Community and Teaching Hospital, however, citations have no independent effect on rank when the other variables are controlled, while their effect at University Hospital and Research Center is quite large.[10] Conversely, productivity has much less of

---

[10] Those who have examined the above partial correlations carefully will have noticed two things which may appear questionable, at least on the surface. First, the fourth-order partial correlation between age and rank for the sample as a whole was .32, and for the two institutions separately they are .32 and .29. These values are possible because the number of cases for Community and Teaching Hospital is significantly less than that for University Hospital (96 vs. 486).

Secondly, the dramatic drop in the partial correlation between citations and rank for Community and Teaching Hospital could be due to an equally dramatic drop in the variance in citations at that institution. While the variance does drop to about half that for the sample as a whole, it remains at 154 and is, therefore, still quite large. The mean number of citations at Community and Teaching Hospital is 6.5.

an independent effect on rank at University Hospital than it does at Community Hospital. Also, seniority has an enhanced effect at Community Hospital while it has less of an effect at University Hospital. It is clear that University Hospital and Research Center does much better at discriminating quality of research output from mere quantity, while at Community and Teaching Hospital no distinction seems to be made on the basis of quality of output. Publishing scientific papers seems to be sufficient as a basis of reward at Community Hospital whereas it is not at University Hospital.

What are the implications for ethical practices of working within the kind of local-institutional reward system we have just described? Crucial for our argument is the assumption that researchers know that the criteria for achievement of rank that we have just analyzed do operate in their institutions. From their knowledge of other organizations as well as from what they have observed of the careers of others and of their own, our researchers should not be surprised if we presented the foregoing relationships to them. Furthermore, we also assume that they will be aware of it if, in comparison with their colleagues, they have not been rewarded with rank in a manner commensurate with their level on the specified bases of local reward. Given these assumptions, we would expect those who are underrewarded in any respect to feel deprived and to want to do something about it, perhaps by raising their level on one of the several bases of rank. For many, publication of scientific papers may offer an easy route to this goal. And, because taking advantage of human subjects can produce better data more certainly and quicker, engaging in a study with a less favorable risks-benefits ratio may be viewed in some quarters as effective for this purpose.

We propose, then, to compare the actual practices, as measured by our two risks-benefits ratios, of researchers who have been underrewarded when their level is taken into account on four of the bases of institutional rank that we have analyzed (citations, productivity, age, and seniority) with the practices of researchers who have not been underrewarded. Therapeutic consults will not be analyzed for the reasons mentioned earlier.

Our measures of fairness of local-institutional reward were all developed in the same way. Because the two institutions studied vary in their reward structures, researchers' rewards were compared only with those of others in their own institution. The rank structures in the two institutions were identical, and so rank was collapsed into three convenient categories: research fellow or less, assistant attending physician, and associate attending physician or higher. Tenure comes only with an appointment to associate attending, and full membership on the senior staff comes only with appointment to the rank of assistant attending, so the cutting points have important meaning for organizational functioning and individual prestige. A researcher was judged underrewarded on the quality of research dimension if he was at one of the two lower ranks and had more citations to his work than the median number for those researchers in his institution at the rank above him. Similarly, underrewardedness on the age, seniority, and productivity dimensions was determined by comparison with the median for the rank above.

Let us now see whether being underrewarded in the sense in which we have defined it is at all related to participating in studies with unfavorable risks-benefits ratios. Table 5.4 relates all four "fairness of local reward" vari-

Table 5.4. Fairness of Local Rewards for Age, Seniority, Productivity, and Research Quality by Risks-Benefits Ratio for Subjects

Fairness of Local Rewards for:	Per Cent Involved in Less Favorable Studies	
	Under rewarded	Rewarded
Age	31% (48)	18% (519)
Seniority	30% (44)	18% (523)
Productivity	20% (94)	19% (473)
Research quality (Citations)	25% (64)	18% (503)

ables to the Risks-Benefits Ratio for Subjects, in which only therapeutic benefit to present subjects is considered.[11] While there is certainly some tendency in the expected direction, the differences are not large, and there were no differences at all using the Risks–All Benefits Ratio. We need to look a little farther.

We felt it was possible that the underrewarded categories in these variables have not sufficiently isolated those groups of researchers who actually "feel" relatively deprived. Knowing that you are underrewarded and actually feeling relatively deprived are both essential, we have hypothesized, to the motivation to participate in studies with less favorable risks-benefits ratios. For example, we wondered if researchers who were trained in elite medical schools,[12] the faculty of which are highly involved in research, might

---

[11] We switch to tabular analysis here because the effects we are going to describe are the result of interactions.

[12] American medical schools were classified as "elite" or "nonelite" by us on the basis of a rating by physicians which was reported in Carol Schwartz, "Schools of Thought in Psychoanalysis: A Study in the Sociology of Knowledge" (unpublished Ph.D. dissertation, Dept. of Sociology, Yale University, 1969), p. 155. Schwartz's raters were all from one Eastern medical school and, though we and she would have preferred a rating by a representative sample of academic physicians or by the deans of the medical schools themselves, no such study was available. The elite medical schools category in Schwartz's scale did not include any West Coast schools, a possible bias according to the opinions of some, but not of importance to us since hardly any of our respondents went to medical

not feel much more personally involved with the high-quality research enterprise than those who were trained either in nonelite American schools or in foreign schools. In addition, we assumed, such men should certainly expect their elite training to pay off in a higher success rate than those with other training.[13] Conversely, those who were trained at nonelite schools and who now find themselves with appointments at an elite university hospital and research center are likely to feel somewhat rewarded already. Thus, when they are underrewarded in regard to their research quality, it should have a smaller psychological effect. Table 5.5 lends some support to this kind

Table 5.5. Per Cents Engaged in Less Favorable and Least Favorable Studies by Quality of Medical School and Fairness of Local Reward for Research Quality (Citations)

Per Cent Engaged in Less Favorable Studies

Fairness of Local Reward for Research Quality	*Quality of Medical School*	
	Elite	*Nonelite or Foreign*
Underrewarded	36% (31)[a]	5% (19)
Rewarded	20% (249)	14% (248)

Per Cent Engaged in Least Favorable Studies

Underrewarded	19% (31)	0% (19)
Rewarded	7% (249)	6% (248)

[a] + 11% when compared to Table 5.4.

of social psychological analysis. Those researchers who were underrewarded when their research quality (citations) is taken into account and who also went to elite medical schools do show a tendency to participate more frequently in studies with less favorable risks-benefits ratios.

The problem of extreme mass producers also came to mind in this connection. In the last chapter we analyzed mechanisms by which extreme mass

---

school on the West Coast. Medical schools classified as elite on this scale were, in alphabetical order: Albert Einstein College of Medicine, Case Western Reserve, University of Chicago, Columbia, Cornell, Duke, Emory, Harvard, Johns Hopkins, New York University, North Carolina, Pennsylvania, University of Rochester, Washington University of St. Louis, and Yale.

[13] Being from an elite medical school is correlated .15 with rank in our two institutions, but this relationship disappears when quality of research, quantity of research, age and seniority are taken into account.

producers seemed to be led into engaging in studies with less favorable risks-benefits ratios. We described them as striving hard but unsuccessfully for recognition from the larger scientific community. They had produced more than ten scientific papers in the previous five years, but had received no citations whatsoever to any of the work they had done. We saw them as being spurred on to even greater efforts by this lack of competitive success, efforts which included more frequent participation in studies with unfavorable risks-benefits ratios for the subjects involved.

What if, we therefore thought, in addition to their lack of national recognition, extreme mass producers were also underrewarded in their local institutions for their productivity? We have seen above that in both of our institutions productivity is independently related to rank, though much more so in Community and Teaching Hospital. Extreme mass producers, being highly productive, ought to be able to expect *some* local recognition even if national recognition in the form of citations eluded them. Table 5.6

Table 5.6   Per Cents Engaged in Less Favorable and Least Favorable Studies by Quality-Quantity Typology and Fairness of Local Reward for High Productivity

Per Cent Engaged in Less Favorable Studies				
Fairness of Local Reward for High Productivity	*Quality-Quantity Typology*			
	High Quality	*Moderate Mass Producers*	*Extreme Mass Producers*	*Silent Scientists*
Underrewarded	23% (35)	4% (23)	53% (17)[a]	5% (19)
Rewarded	19% (145)	21% (43)	25% (8)	18% (271)

Per Cent Engaged in Least Favorable Studies				
Underrewarded	6% (35)	0% (23)	29% (17)[b]	5% (19)
Rewarded	8% (145)	12% (43)	0% (8)	6% (271)

[a] + 14% when compared to Table 4.7.
[b] + 11% when compared to Table 4.7.

shows the effect on rates of involvement by extreme mass producers in less favorable studies when they are also underrewarded in their local institutions for their productivity. Though the small number of cases involved indicates that we should be cautious, the differences are highly suggestive. It is also in the nature of things that there cannot be many extreme mass producers or underrewarded researchers using criteria as extreme as the ones we have set up. They are of necessity deviant types in a system which does reward merit and service and does discourage the existence of mass producers by failing to recognize their work or reward it by citations.

So far we have examined those types of researchers who seem to be working hardest at achieving rank by being high on quality or quantity of scientific work. We have presented some evidence that researchers from elite medical schools who were underrewarded when the quality of their work was taken into account were more frequently involved in studies with unfavorable risks-benefit ratios. And just now we looked at extreme mass producers who were underrewarded when their high productivity is taken into account. What about the case of relative nonproducers, that is, what the Coles called the silent scientists. Their relatively low involvement in research, as evidenced by both lower average productivity and lower number of ongoing research projects, is an indication that they probably do not view success in research as their means to higher local institutional rank. Perhaps they are attempting to succeed locally by being recognized as highly competent therapists or administrators. There is, unfortunately, no way for us to be sure. It should be the case, however, that they, more than the other types in our Quality-Quantity Typology, should feel deprived if they are underrewarded when their age or seniority is taken into account. By not achieving in the research area, they essentially forsake the possibility of a really rapid rise in the institution and hope for due recognition of long and faithful service. And, as Table 5.7 shows, silent scientists do form a much

Table 5.7. Proportion of Those Who Are At All Locally Underrewarded Who Fall into the Four Quality-Quantity Types (percentaged by row)

Locally Underrewarded by:	Quality-Quantity Typology				
	High Quality	Moderate Mass Producers	Extreme Mass Producers	Silent Scientists	
Seniority	21%	9	0	70	100% (44)
Age	27%	0	10	63	100% (48)
Productivity	37%	25	18	20	100% (94)
Research quality (Citations)	72%	13	0	15	100% (64)

higher proportion of those who are underrewarded according to age and seniority than they do of those who are underrewarded when quality or quantity of research is taken into account.

If the pattern of our analysis holds, we should expect silent scientists who are underrewarded when their age or seniority is considered to partic- ipate more frequently in studies with less favorable risks-benefits ratios. By producing publishable research, our argument goes, they may thereby be trying to assure the promotion that mere longevity and faithful service have not provided. The data in Table 5.8, using the Risks-Benefits Ratio

Table 5.8   Per Cents Engaged in Less Favorable Studies by Fairness of Local Rewards for Age and for Seniority by Quality-Quantity Typology

Per Cents Engaged in Less Favorable Studies				
	Quality-Quantity Typology			
Fairness of Local Reward for Age	*High Quality*	*Moderate Mass Producers*	*Extreme Mass Producers*	*Silent Scientists*
Underrewarded	15% (13)	— (0)	— (5)	37% (30)
Rewarded	20% (167)	15% (66)	45% (20)	15% (260)
Fairness of Local Reward for Seniority				
Underrewarded	11% (9)	— (4)	— (0)	39% (31)
Rewarded	20% (171)	16% (62)	44% (25)	15% (259)

for Subjects, are suggestive in this regard, though it must be pointed out that the differences are minimal if the Risks–All Benefits Ratio is used. In Table 5.8 silent scientists who are underrewarded for age or seniority are more likely to be involved in studies where the Risks-Benefits Ratio for Subjects is less favorable for the subjects.

We have shown in this chapter that the reward systems in the two local institutions we have studied are multidimensional. Other things being equal, we see, researchers can achieve higher rank in a number of different ways. We have also suggested that researchers make choices as to the means of achieving rank they will emphasize. Some do it by striving hard to produce publishable research which they hope will be of high quality. Others hope that their therapeutic or administrative competence, their seniority, or their institutional loyalty, will be recognized, and they rely on the institution to reward service to it rather than to science in general. Our data show further that those who have been less rewarded by local rank than peers for whatever they have performed in the area they have emphasized, are more likely to be led to take advantage of human subjects in order to increase their chances of promotion by publishing significant scientific work.

It is unfortunate that we have relatively few cases of underrewarded researchers from Community and Teaching Hospital as compared to University Hospital and Research Center because of the interesting differences

between their local reward systems. One would expect that the various processes leading to doing more permissive studies would operate differently in
the two institutions as a function of the differences in reward systems, but
we are unfortunately unable to explore these possibilities.

Our data suggest, then, that not only does the social structure of scientific competition and reward in the larger scientific community seem to lead
to negative consequences for human subjects, so also does competition for
rank of various kinds at the local-institutional level. We see again the dilemma of science and therapy. Both are important values and can often be
satisfactorily adjusted one to the other. But the dilemma of science and
therapy is not satisfactorily resolved when objective failure or feelings of
unfairness in either the larger or the local-institutional scientific reward systems exert pressure upon the researcher to put science ahead of humane
therapy and to adopt the more permissive rather than the more strict pattern
of behavior.

6

SOCIAL CONTROL: SOME PATTERNS
AND CONSEQUENCES OF SOCIALIZATION

We turn now from our first explanatory variable, the conflict of equal values in socially structured situations, to our second one, the structures and processes of social control. In the previous two chapters we have seen how, in this biomedical research instance of value-conflict, the dilemma of science and therapy interacts with the competition structures of science to produce certain patterns of ethical conformity and deviance. Now, similarly, we wish to show how various social control structures and processes also contribute to determining these patterns.

Among sociologists, the concept of social control is construed quite broadly and includes structures and processes which are both formal and informal, both manifest and latent. It is used to refer to many diverse structures and processes, of which we shall study only three. First, it refers to those structures and processes that instill the knowledge, values, norms, and ideologies into social actors that they need to carry on or innovate in their roles. This first type of social control, which is often called socialization, is what we shall report on in this chapter. Social control includes, second, those structures and processes that bring the pressures of informal social interaction to bear on behalf of conformity or deviance. In the next chapter we shall inquire how scientific collaboration groups and other informal interaction networks may affect the strict and permissive patterns we have discerned among biomedical researchers. Third and finally, social control also includes the structures and processes for applying the several rewards and punishments that various private and governmental organizations have defined as necessary for producing desirable social performance in any given sphere. In later chapters, when we discuss the patterns and consequences of ethical peer review, we shall be looking at this type of social control of biomedical researchers. In sum, social control is what produces the mixture of conformity and deviance in society, the balance of order and disorder. In the rest of the book it will be our main independent or explanatory variable.

In this chapter, then, we are interested in one aspect of the ethical socialization of biomedical researchers, namely, those structures, processes, and experiences which are supposed to instill in them the knowledge, values, and norms necessary for satisfactory ethical performance with regard to the use of human subjects. We shall proceed by first reporting the methods and instruments we used to collect our data in this area. Then we shall describe a developmental sequence of socialization experiences, structures, and processes through which biomedical researchers pass, from premedical school experiences to the structures and processes of medical school, internship and residency, and research groups themselves. Then we shall show how our data on a few of the patterns produced by the stages of this sequence have some consequences for at least the expressed standards of biomedical researchers with regard to the consent and the risk-benefit issues. Our data do not show any effects of socialization structures and processes *by themselves* on conformity or deviance in respect to actual behavior in research using human subjects. However, socialization patterns, when taken *together with* certain informal interaction and authority patterns, do seem to have such effects. The discussion of the effects produced by this interaction of socialization, on the one hand, with informal interaction and authority structures, on the other, will be reserved for the next chapter, where we will need first to describe some of these latter structures.

DATA AND METHODS

It will be recalled from Chapter 2, where we gave our general discussion of methodology, that our data on socialization structures and processes were collected by personal interview in our second study, the Intensive Two-Institution Study. In that study we interviewed 352 biomedical researchers in person and obtained responses to shortened mailed questionnaires from 35 more. Researchers at University Hospital and Research Center made up 298 of the personal interviews while 54 were conducted at Community and Teaching Hospital. Since physicians constitute the larger majority of our researcher-respondents, and since the importance of medical school and clinical training in socialization is clear from the data, in this chapter we deal with only the 307 researchers in the study who are physicians. In reading the following discussion, it should be kept firmly in mind that the data here are "retrospective," that is, that the respondents were asked to recall past experiences and feelings.

Because there were no models for our study, that is, not a single previous investigation of the specific socialization patterns in which we were interested, the majority of the questions in this section of the interview schedule were open-ended and exploratory. Hence, we were unable to include them in the shortened mailed questionnaire which was completed by the 35 additional researchers mentioned above. In future studies, more specific questions will be easier to construct. There were, then, three types of questions.[1]

The first type dealt with the salience of socialization experiences. Respondents were asked to recall their first awareness of the ethical issues discussed earlier in the interview, that is, their first awareness of the necessity and difficulty of assessing the potential risk and potential benefit of any research procedure, and their first awareness of the conditions under which the informed consent of research subjects was appropriate. They were also asked what experience had been most important in the development of their present attitudes toward these issues.

The second type of question probed for recall of experiences which had made the respondent aware of the ethical issues at crucial points in his development as a researcher—before medical school, during medical school, during internship and residency, and at the beginning of his research career.

The third type of question dealt with the presence or absence of specific experiences which were suggested in the literature on medical training as having an impact on ethical formation: being the subject of research, doing research with human subjects during medical school, having discussions with other medical students or working with experimental animals, reading any of the discussions of research ethics available, and having had formal courses or seminars in research ethics. Researchers were asked to recall whether they had had such experiences and their reactions to them.[2]

It will also be recalled from Chapter 2 that, because of the time constraints of our personal interviews with researchers and because of the very large amount of time it had taken respondents to our National Survey to give answers to our six research protocols dealing with the consent and risk-benefit issues, we had reduced these protocols to two in our second study. By choosing the two that we had discovered in the first study to be most comprehensive in their coverage of the two issues and to be most productive of a range of responses, we needed only to alter one of them slightly to have satisfactory measures for our dependent variables with regard to expressed standards (see Appendix II). Responses to these two hypothetical questions are the measures used in this and the next chapters. So far as actual behavior is concerned, of course, we have used the reports about estimated risk and benefit that our respondents in this second study gave us. Response to the

---

[1] See questions 18 to 29, Appendix II.

[2] Those descriptions of training and research settings which were most useful were Renée C. Fox, *Experiment Perilous* (Glencoe, Ill.: Free Press, 1959); Renée C. Fox, "A Sociological Calendar of Medical School" (unpublished, 1958); Robert K. Merton, George G. Reader, and Patricia L. Kendall, eds., *The Student Physician* (Cambridge, Mass.: Harvard University Press, 1957); Stephen Miller, *Prescription for Leadership* (Chicago: Aldine, 1970).

two protocols and self-reports on behavior are our two measures, then, of the dependent variables, the effects on which of socialization we are trying to discover.

Another, more general "methodological" point needs to be emphasized here. It should constantly be kept in mind that neither the processes of socialization in general and certainly not those relevant for biomedical research are as well understood or as satisfactorily researched as they might be.[3] Socialization processes are themselves complex, developmental, and not readily made more effective. Certainly, because socialization often interacts with other determinants of concrete behavior, we cannot say that "poor socialization" is the sole cause of deviance. While better knowledge and better values can probably be better instilled by improved socialization processes, "knowledge" alone is no solution for ethical problems in this area. Codes help and knowledge of codes helps, but more is needed. Keeping these cautions in mind will be useful as we discuss socialization.

THE SEQUENTIAL STAGES OF ETHICAL SOCIALIZATION

Before proceeding to an account of what our respondents told us happened in each of the several stages of socialization, let us look at some data which will tell us at what time during the socialization sequence respondents report that they were first aware of the ethical issues involved in research with human subjects. The first question in the socialization section of the interview schedule was, "Can you remember when you first became aware

---

[3] For something of what is known about socialization in general from the perspective used here, see the several essays in John A. Clausen, ed., *Socialization and Society* (Boston: Little, Brown, 1968). For the socialization of physicians, though with no special emphasis on research, see Robert K. Merton, et al., *The Student Physician.* In an appendix Merton presents a history and analysis of the use of the term "socialization." See also Eliot Freidson's excellent book, *Profession of Medicine* (New York: Dodd Mead, 1970). Although, in general, Freidson tends to minimize the importance of socialization as compared with "work-context" in determining professional behavior, he says at one point (p. 88), "There is no question at all that the education in attitude and skill that the physician obtains in medical school and in the hospital where he is an intern and resident is an *absolute* source of much of his performance as a practitioner." Further data on professional socialization, most of it inconclusive as to its effects, can be found in Jerome Carlin, *Lawyers' Ethics: A Survey of the New York City Bar* (New York: Russell Sage Foundation, 1966), pp. 143–145. Finally, see Jay Katz, "The Education of the Physician-Investigator," *Daedalus* (Spring, 1969): 480–501.

In general, it is our theoretical position that socialization and "work-context" are two independent variables which work sometimes independently, sometimes interdependently. In general, it needs to be seen in sociological analysis that variables in a system are, in principle, both independent in some measure and also interdependent. It is an empirical problem, then, to measure the amounts of independence and interdependence.

of the issues involved in the use of human subjects in research?" The responses are given in Table 6.1, which makes clear several interesting facts we shall explore more fully later. First, only 17% of the sample came to medical school aware of an aspect of medicine which is important to both researchers and practitioners; they were the only ones who might use their

Table 6.1. Time at Which Physician-Investigators First Became Aware of the Ethical Issues of Human Experimentation

Before medical school	17%
During medical school	41
During clinical training	13
During research career	29
	100% (307)

earlier awareness as a base for further socialization in medical school. Second, even at the end of medical school training, 42% of our sample still were not aware of the ethical problems of using human subjects in research. And, third, despite this earlier failure of socialization to occur, there is, further, a considerable amount of "on the job" ethical training for researchers, first in their clinical training and then in actual research work itself. Now let us look at the several stages individually.

EXPERIENCES BEFORE MEDICAL SCHOOL

Our second question in the socialization set asked, "Did you have any experiences before medical school which made you aware of the issues involved in the use of human subjects in research?" Table 6.2 provides a summary of the experiences reported in answer to this question. In collapsing the ninety response categories for presentation in the descriptive tables for each stage in the socialization sequence, two criteria were used.[4] First, each category or group of related categories which includes more than ten respondents' answers has been presented in the table. Second, each category which includes only a few responses at a given time, but which represents responses which will be used for analysis because of their cumulative interest or importance at a later time has been included in the table. An example of a category of little importance before medical school is awareness of the

---

[4] The complete list of categories used in coding the responses to the open-ended questions is included in Julia Loughlin Makarushka, "Learning to be Ethical: Patterns of Socialization and Their Variable Consequences for the Ethical Standards of Bio-Medical Researchers" (Unpublished dissertation, Columbia University, 1971), Appendix III.

Table 6.2.   Types of Experiences That Made Physician-Investigators Aware of the Ethical Issues of Research before Medical School

None	67%ª
Learned about general ethical issues from nonfiction	9
Learned about Nazi experiments	6
Discussed research ethics with others	4
Learned about research which made aware of ethical problems	4
Was the subject of biomedical or psychological research	2
Saw others benefiting from, or in need of, knowledge gained from research	1
Other	7
	100% (307)

ª This figure is smaller than one would expect from the previous table because, when asked the second question, some of our respondents who had said "not before medical school" on the first question, now mentioned some premedical school experience.

benefits or necessity of research advances. Only three respondents report such awareness before medical school but, as we shall see later, such a response during medical school seems to represent a distinctive orientation toward biomedical research.

The fact that the reading of nonfiction is the most frequent response indicates the importance of books, newspapers, and the other communication media as socializing agents for eventual researchers and, probably also, for the general public. The single event that is mentioned most frequently, the Nazi experimentation on unconsenting human subjects in concentration camps during World War II, further confirms this importance.[5] Awareness of the concentration camp horrors was hard to avoid. The events occurred during the lifetime of most respondents, they were very highly publicized, and they occasioned perhaps the best-known and most widely distributed of all codes of research ethics, the Nuremberg Code. The reaction to these experiments by those who reported awareness of them was, of course, negative. Widespread publicity has been given to many other research advances in medicine, and of all "science" news, that connected with medicine is the most widely read by the general public. In *Experiment Perilous*, where Renée Fox has described the research groups that first did research on such problems as treatment with cortisone, the usefulness of total adrenalectomies, and the feasibility of the first kidney transplants, she describes the press

[5] See United States Adjutant General's Department, *Trials of War Criminals Before Nuremberg Military Tribunals Under Control Council Law No. 10* (Oct., 1946–April, 1947), *The Medical Case* (Washington, D.C.: U.S. Government Printing Office, 1947).

coverage of the experimental drugs and procedures "the Metabolic Group" pioneered.[6] More recently, she has given an account of the publicity that has been given to the development of mitral valve surgery. In this case, Fox notes that

> the content of all the news articles we have examined . . . is highly positive and triumphant in tone. Valvular surgery is presented as a harbinger of a new era of open heart surgery, and emphasis is placed on the "new life" that such operations can make possible for former cardiac invalids.[7]

But triumph can turn to pessimism and even despair, as has recently been manifest in newspaper, magazine, and other publicity about heart transplants. The diverse socializing effects of media publicity on eventual researchers, eventual patients, and the general public needs further scrutiny.

In sum, with regard to the period before they began their medical training, about two-thirds of our respondents reported no awareness at all of the issues involved in the use of human subjects in experimentation. But even such awareness was not uniform in its effects. Those who did become aware of these matters this early on were about evenly divided between those who were aware of some serious abuse of the rights or welfare of the subjects of research and those who said they first saw the problems in the light of a generally favorable view of the biomedical research enterprise. Such differences in first awareness may have their effects later.

EXPERIENCES DURING MEDICAL SCHOOL

Medical schools have probably been more studied than any other type of professional education. The medical school curriculum is continually under review as new fields, new problems, and new emphases compete for attention. As Robert Merton pointed out in *The Student-Physician*, the medical student is socialized not only in the classroom but also in continuing interaction with instructors, peers, patients, and nurses, and acquires not only a vast amount of knowledge and skill, but also the appropriate attitudes, values, and behavior patterns.[8]

In an unpublished report dealing with the first two years of medical school, Renée Fox has summarized some findings of an intensive qualitative study that was designed to complement the Student-Physician questionnaire. She used systematic observations, extensive interviews, and diaries kept by

---

[6] Fox, *op. cit.*, pp. 145–147.

[7] Judith P. Swazey and Renée C. Fox, "The Clinical Moratorium: A Case Study of Mitral Valve Surgery," in Paul A. Freund, ed., *Experimentation With Human Subjects* (New York: George Braziller, 1970), p. 343.

[8] Merton, "Some Preliminaries . . . ," pp. 41–42.

twelve of the eighty students in a class of students at one medical school to develop a picture of the patterned processes by which the students were socialized. Here emphasis was not on their learning of facts through formal lectures and reading, but on the development of values and attitudes, particularly an attitude of "detached concern" for patients, and on the ability to deal with the inevitable uncertainty involved in medicine. Fox stresses the ways in which the students developed group norms and provided social support for one another. She also illuminates the unsystematic as well as systematic processes of socialization into norms and values.[9]

Probably because there was so little attention to the problem in medical circles when Merton, Fox, and their colleagues were doing their work (only 20 years ago), training in the ethics of experimenting with humans was not an explicit focus of attention in their study, but several types of experiences common in the first two years of medical school were nevertheless noted as incidentally alerting some students to these ethical problems. First, in performing experiments with animals, students were explicitly taught the necessity of justifying the animals' suffering, even their deaths, by "getting everything possible" out of the experiment. Fox suggests that such experiences with animals would help the students to deal with their own feelings when faced in practice with the conflict between research and therapy.[10]

Second, she suggests, in doing experiments on one another in physiology lab, second-year students were exposed to two principles of research ethics: the rule that an investigator should not ask his human subjects to participate in any experiment which he would not perform on himself, and the rule that in an experiment involving risk, the subject must be protected by the "constant surveillance of the researcher." An emphasis on the students' obligation to submit to experimentation is implied in the instructor's discussion of these experiments, as well as other experiments and practice procedures, but there is nowhere any mention of the right not to submit; or of the right to be fully informed of the purpose of the experimental procedures and their anticipated outcomes.[11]

Third, an incident in the second year precipitated a vigorous discussion among the students of informed consent, the "usual" practice in research. A special lecturer on nutrition presented, apparently without ethical comment, data from a study of malnutrition conducted without consent with Korean

---

[9] Renée C. Fox, "A Sociological Calendar of the First Year in Medical School" (unpublished, 1958) and "A Sociological Calendar of Medical School: Second Year, First Trimester" (unpublished, 1956).

[10] Fox, "A Sociological Calendar of Medical School," pp. 21, 51, and Fox, "A Sociological Calendar of the First Year . . . ," p. 124.

[11] Fox, "A Sociological Calendar of Medical School," pp. 77–78, 21–22 and Fox, "A Sociological Calendar of the First Year . . . ," pp. 107–109, 124.

prisoners of war. The students, in their discussion, referred not to medical research ethics, but to more general standards:

> . . . in the mind of the (reporting) student and some of his classmates such experiments on human subjects, whether prisoners-of-war or otherwise are "immoral" as measured against the values of the "American Creed" in which they were "brought up to believe."[12]

These preliminary but insightful data from Fox's work suggested to us that experiences connected with work with animals, with practice procedures, with being the subject of biomedical research, with discussions with fellow-students or teachers, and with work read about or learned of in class were potentially or latently socializing experiences, though not explicitly intended to teach the principles of research ethics.

Because of Fox's suggestions about the probably unintended effects of these medical school experiences, we decided to collect some systematic evidence about them. Therefore, all respondents interviewed for the Two-Institution Study were asked if, in fact, they had become aware of the two issues of risk versus benefits or the necessity of obtaining informed consent as a result of such experiences. In addition, we asked each respondent if he had had a course or seminar in medical school which dealt explicitly with the issues of risk and consent in human experimentation.

It is clear from our data that medical schools are presently giving very little serious attention to these matters in their curriculum. Of the 307 physicians interviewed, only 13% reported that they had had a seminar, a lecture or part of a course devoted to the issues involved in the use of human subjects in biomedical research, and only one researcher said that he had had a complete course dealing with these issues. Thirteen per cent of the respondents said that the issues of research ethics came up when as students they did practice procedures on one another, and 24% said that they became aware of the issues of balancing risk or suffering against potential benefits when doing experimental work with animals. Thirty-four per cent remembered discussions with instructors or other students of the ethical issues involved in specific research projects which they had read about or learned of in class. But 57% of the physicians interviewed reported none of these experiences, even those peripheral to work with humans, such as those involving animal experimentation.

Even work with humans, our data show, does not necessarily socialize medical students into the ethical problems of research. Nineteen per cent of the respondents reported that they had conducted some research with human subjects while they were in medical school, but of these 59 respondents,

---

[12] Fox, "A Sociological Calendar of Medical School . . . ," p. 23.

only 31 reported that ethical issues had ever been considered in the course of such research.

Nor does serving as a subject oneself necessarily socialize one into ethical concerns. The majority of those who themselves served as research subjects *at any time* in the course of their training or own research careers reported that such an experience did not in any way make them aware of the ethical issues involved in human experimentation. Moreover as Table 6.3 shows,

Table 6.3. Reaction to Having Been the Subject of Biomedical Experimentation

	At Any Time	During Medical School
No increased awareness	51%	51%
Increased awareness of risk or consent	35	40
Understanding of the subject's feelings	12	7
Awareness of the value of research	2	2
	100% (240)	100% (122)

when respondents were subjects during their medical school years, they were not more likely to have become aware of the ethical problems, as a result, than those who served as subjects either earlier or later in their careers.

After we asked these questions probing for specific experiences during medical school, the physician-researchers were asked an open-ended question: "Was there any other experience during medical school which made you aware of the issues involved in the use of human subjects of research?" An additional experience was mentioned in answer to this question by 104 respondents, about one-third of the total sample. The experiences most frequently mentioned are summarized in Table 6.4.

The types of experiences mentioned, of course, reflect the new kinds of experience to which the medical student is exposed—teachers actively engaged in research, access to a wider body of research literature, and the research subjects themselves among the patients in a teaching hospital.

The category "aware through teachers' concern" includes those responses which indicated that specific teachers had either specifically emphasized relevant values or norms, or had provided models of ethical research through their example in their relationship with their own subjects. The category "aware of responsibility as a physician" includes those responses which emphasized the students' understanding that they were responsible for their patients' well-being, that they were enjoined to "do no harm."

Table 6.4.   Types of Other Experiences Which Made Physician-Investigators Aware of the Ethical Issues of Research during Medical School

None	66%
Aware of responsibility as a physician	8
Aware through teachers' concern	7
Saw the need for further research	5
Learned about research which raised ethical questions	4
Became aware of subjects' negative reactions to research	3
Other	7
	100% (303)

It is significant that younger respondents in our sample are more likely to report experiences in medical school than are older respondents. On the one hand, the increase in the amount of research being done in the past twenty years, and the increased concern with possible controls to insure the protection of the rights and welfare of the subjects of research would lead one to expect that there would have been an increase in the extent to which medical students would be exposed to the ethics of biomedical research either formally and deliberately or informally, through the example of their instructors or exposure to one of the many discussions of research ethics published since 1950. On the other hand, we cannot be sure that some of the failure to report experiences among our older respondents is not due simply to the longer time that has passed since their graduation from medical school and consequent difficulty in remembering such experiences. Two facts lead us to attribute at least part of the tendency of the younger respondents to report more experiences to the actual existence of an increased emphasis on research ethics among biomedical researchers in particular and other members of the medical school faculty in general. First, many of our older respondents recognized and explicitly stated that the situation had changed, that research ethics were simply not mentioned during their time at medical school, that students then would not have felt able to question an instructor's judgment or raise a controversial point for discussion, but that "things are different now." Second, the differences are greatest between those who graduated before 1950 and those after 1950. Those who graduated between 1950 and 1960, twenty to ten years ago, are very similar in the number of experiences they report to those who graduated more recently. We would expect failing memories to operate to produce a more gradual change. Table 6.5 shows the differences in the number of explicit medical school socialization experiences (courses dealing with research ethics, at least in part, practice procedures or work with animals in which research ethics are brought up, discussions with others of specific research projects which raised

Table 6.5.   Year of Graduation from Medical School by Number of Formal
Socializing Experiences in Medical School

Number of Experiences	Before 1950	1950– 1959	1960– present	Total
None	63%	43%	33%	44%
One	28	34	42	35
Two or three	9	23	25	21
Totals	100% (72)	100% (121)	100% (108)	100% (301)
	24%	40%	36%	100%

ethical questions) reported by respondents graduating from medical schools
at different times.

The type of medical school attended seems to make no difference in the
number of socializing experiences to which medical students are exposed.
There are no differences in the frequency with which each kind of experience is mentioned by graduates of elite American medical schools, other
American medical schools, or foreign medical schools. This uniformity further indicates how widespread is the lack of serious training in these ethical
problems in the medical schools.

SOCIALIZATION EXPERIENCES DURING INTERNSHIP AND RESIDENCY

The years of clinical training are crucial to the career development of
the young biomedical researcher. During the three to five years of internship
and residency he acquires the experience in dealing with problems which he
has come to value so highly.[13] He tests his ability and his satisfaction with
his chosen profession and demonstrates his competence to those who will
help him in the next stage of his career.

We did not ask our respondents at which hospitals they served as interns and residents. Most of them, however, would have served at institutions
similar to our University Hospital and Research Center, since it is from such

---

[13] The importance of practical experience to validate or even contradict "textbook
knowledge" is stressed by Howard S. Becker, *et al., Boys in White* (Chicago: University
of Chicago Press, 1962), ch. 12, and by Freidson, *Profession of Medicine*, pp. 166, 347.
Freidson notes that "much of the practical knowledge of the profession is based on personal clinical experience. Indeed, much of the scientific knowledge of medicine stems from
individual discoveries by great individual clinicians, and the model of the clinician still
so dominates the everyday practices and ideology of medicine as to encourage individual
deviation from codified knowledge on the basis of personal, firsthand observation of
concrete cases" (p. 347).

institutions that researchers are selected.[14] It is in the internship and residency years that the young investigator begins to be actively involved in research, either on some relatively small research project under the guidance of the head of the department, or as a subordinate in some major research project. Such research, perhaps some first publications, is necessary for entry into and promotion in institutions like University Hospital and Research Center. As Henry Beecher has noted,

> Medical schools and university hospitals are increasingly dominated by investigators. Every young physician knows that he will never be promoted to a tenure post, to a professorship in a major medical school, unless he has proven himself as an investigator. If the ready availability of money for conducting research is added to this fact, one can see how great are the pressures on ambitious young physicians.[15]

Two-thirds of our respondents who described themselves as "ever seriously active in research" had become active before the end of their residency. They were not necessarily independent researchers at this point, but frequently worked with others. The experiences described in this section are in answer to the question "Did any of these issues with respect to human subjects come up in some new way in your *clinical experience* during your internship or residency years?" If our respondents viewed the experience during the period of internship and residency as related to their position as physicians in training it is included in this section. If a similar experience during the same time period, internship and residency, was seen as related to the respondent's beginning his own independent research it is included in the next section. Table 6.6. summarizes the experiences reported by our respondents during internship and residency.

We can see several changes in the types of socializing experiences to which our respondents have been exposed during these years as against the medical school years. A few more respondents report being troubled by the conflict between the novice doctor's need to learn and the patients' right to receive the best care. They view "practicing on" the patient as a type of experimentation. There is also an increase in the number reporting an awareness of the necessity of research and awareness of subjects who have suffered

---

[14] See Stephen Miller, *Prescription for Leadership*, for an analysis of the recruitment and training of academic physicians. William A. Nolen, in *The Making of a Surgeon* (New York: Random House, 1968), pp. 143–147, provides an interesting example of a resident who chose the "wrong" residency for entry into an academic career and attempted to rectify his mistake by quickly producing some research publications. This case dramatizes not only the need for the "correct" choice of residency for entry into research institutions but also the ease with which ward patients may be used as subjects of research in which their interests are not protected.

[15] *Research and the Individual*, p. 14.

Table 6.6.   Types of Experiences Which Made Physician-Investigators Aware of the Ethical Issues of Research during Their Clinical Training

None	41%
Research apprenticeship	23
Learned of research which raised ethical questions	7
Aware of responsibility as a physician	7
Aware through teachers' concern	6
Saw the need for further research	6
Became aware of subjects' negative reactions to research	4
Other	6
	100% (306)

untoward consequences of research procedures. The research projects which alert the interns and residents to ethical problems are no longer research reports in medical journals: 18 of the 20 respondents mentioning such awareness are now referring to cases from their personal knowledge.

Our first category in the table, "Research apprenticeship" includes 23% of our respondents. The specific responses which are included in this category are: having responsibility for patients whom researchers wished to use as subjects (8%), having performed experimental procedures on patients for other researchers which raised ethical questions (8%), and having performed experimental procedures on patients which made the respondent aware that there were ethical problems involved, without necessarily raising such ethical questions at the time (7%). We have called this the research apprenticeship pattern because the new physicians are actively dealing with the ethical problems of balancing risk against benefit and obtaining informed consent from subjects, but they are still subject themselves to the close supervision of senior researchers. The interns and residents are their patients' only physicians, and are responsible for those patients whom their researcher colleagues wish to use as subjects. Those patients will not be asked to become research subjects without their physicians' consent, and the residents are now the physicians in charge for ward patients. The residents are also often the ones who actually administer the experimental drugs or perform the experimental research procedures and who observe and record any positive or negative consequences for the research subjects. From the point of view of the resident, then, the research apprenticeship pattern gives him practice in conducting research and making ethical decisions through his own experience and through the example of other, senior researchers.

For some interns and residents, that is, at least the 23% of those in our study who specifically volunteer these answers to this question, the research apprenticeship increases their awareness of the ethical problems of adequately safeguarding the rights and welfare of the subjects of biomedical research. Some found themselves under pressure to make decisions which they felt were unethical; some refused to do what they thought was wrong and others felt unable to refuse. Several respondents noted that they proposed research which they were not permitted to carry out, or carried out research for which they were criticized. We can see the new researchers learning a more specific set of norms and values through their subordinate position in the research hierarchy.

The research apprenticeship pattern also has functions other than that of training new investigators. It is sometimes a mechanism wherein interns may exchange information and research assistance for the services of senior researchers as consultants and teachers. Stephen Miller has contributed an extensive analysis of this pattern of apprenticeship as exchange in his study of the internship program at the Harvard Medical Unit at Boston City Hospital. In this program and probably elsewhere in research hospital units, not only does the intern obtain consent from patients and perform research procedures, but he also identifies potential subjects for the clinical investigator.

> The consulting physicians are interested in particular kinds of patients for their own reasons, either to further their knowledge or advance their research. Whatever they need patients for, it is almost impossible for them to keep watch for the kinds they need. Interns do this for them. . . . Interns obligate themselves to consulting physicians the first time they seek their help. In exchange for valuable information or services they must furnish the consults with information about patients who might be useful in clinical investigation.[16]

The intern is in principle free not to cooperate, not to identify patients as suitable subjects, or not to agree to the proposed research. This power of refusal places the interns in a position to demand teaching performances from the researchers in return for their own compliance with the researchers' need for subjects. Miller, however, comments that

> I did not once see an intern refuse clinical investigators the permission to use his patients. An intern occasionally complained that the clinical investigators were using his patients as guinea pigs, but he knew that his complaint would not influence those in authority. Interns are, in fact, told that they may not always understand why certain procedures are necessary, or that they may think these things are not in the best interests of their patients. When they have such doubts, they are supposed to consult the clinical investigator. They do not need to be told that any differences of opinion will be resolved in favor of the latter.[17]

---

[16] Stephen Miller, *op. cit.*, pp. 152–153.
[17] *Ibid.*, p. 154.

For ward or clinic patients who are potential subjects, the resident or intern is the only physician; they have no other, private, physician who will advise them when they are asked to be research subjects or who will explain proposed research in the effort to insure their informed consent. Emily Mumford, in her study of internship training, points out the exchange which may take place between the intern and the ward patient:

> In a sense, the exchange of benefits between house staff and ward patient is more even than between the same house-staff member and the private patient on most services. The intern gives service and in return gets to be *the* doctor for the ward patient. The patient provides the chance for learning experience, and sometimes he also agrees to become a research subject in return for the doctor's special interest in him or his medical problem.[18]

Now we can see a little better why, as the data presented in Chapter 3 showed, the least favorable studies are more likely to be done on ward and clinic than on private patients.

SOCIALIZATION EXPERIENCES DURING THE RESEARCH CAREER

After completing his residency, the researcher may have continued being alerted to ethical problems in the course of his own research. Fifty-three per cent of the physicians in the Intensive Two-Institution Study reported that they had some experience during the course of their research career which increased their awareness of the ethical issues of biomedical research. Thirty-nine per cent were reporting experiences which were directly related to their own research: questions of risk or consent arose, researchers were conscious of having the final responsibility for their subjects' welfare, subjects had negative reactions to research procedures, colleagues exerted influence, or formal controls over the use of subjects increased their awareness. Table 6.7 summarizes the types of experiences which were reported as occurring at this time.

As would be expected, there is a decline in the numbers reporting learning from various kinds of experiences which happened to others, or to other researchers' subjects. This is because the investigator now has full responsibility for the decisions made about the amount of risk which is acceptable in a given study and also for the adequacy of the information upon which the subjects will base their consent. He must deal with these ethical problems in a practical, not an abstract way. If he and his subjects are fortunate, he has already been alerted to these problems or he will be alerted by the formal

---

[18] Emily Mumford, *Interns: From Students to Physicians* (Cambridge: Harvard University Press, 1970), p. 30.

Table 6.7.   Types of Experiences Which Made Physician-Investigators Aware of the Ethical Issues of Research during the Research Career

None	47%
Ethical questions arose in own research	19
Own subjects had negative reactions	6
Aware because of increased responsibility	6
Colleagues influenced them	5
Saw the need for further research	4
Became aware of subjects' negative reactions to others' research	4
Formal controls increased awareness	3
Other	6
	100% (307)

control procedures set up to protect the rights and welfare of his subjects. In some cases, however, adequate awareness of the ethical problems of human experimentation followed upon actual harm to the subjects, either unanticipated negative reactions to the research procedures, or the researcher's having been criticized by others for using subjects without their prior knowledge and consent.

While we have no systematic evidence of the consequences of these experiences during their own research for the biomedical researcher's later norms and behavior, some of the comments our respondents volunteered are suggestive. One researcher told us how he had been impressed by the dangers of research:

> Generally, as I have gradually gotten to know the human research field better, I've come to question more the justifiability of much of the human research being done because so much of it is of poor quality and when it is also risky to subjects, it needs to be checked and/or eliminated.

Another told us how so extreme an untoward incident as a patient death had affected him:

> I already had a strong feeling for the patients' concerns and fears from my long clinical experience. A few years ago, I killed a patient during a research procedure: this made me more sensitive to weighing the pros and cons. I was doing catheterization with a new instrument and there were special circumstances. Now, I would not do that experiment.

And another told us of one way he had developed for avoiding the most serious ethical problems:

> The simplest ethical way of doing research on humans is to do research on disease; the risk of the disease is so great, that the ethical problems are small. Keep a medical orientation and stick to patients—a great deal can be learned.

As we have now seen, whether the individual researcher is aware of the ethical issues of experimenting with humans before he begins his own research depends on several factors: his premedical school socializing experiences, and the opportunities presented to him during medical school, internship, and residency. But if he has still not become aware of the issues before his first independent ventures into biomedical research with human subjects, his becoming aware and the specific solutions he chooses for these ethical problems may depend to a great extent on the institution within which the research is conducted.

The importance of the research institution and the research group has been demonstrated by previous research. There are two useful studies of the interaction among members of biomedical research groups engaged in human experimentation as they attempted to find solutions for the ethical dilemmas of human research. The first, *Experiment Perilous*, already referred to, was conducted by Renée Fox. She describes the reaction of investigators and subjects to research conducted in the Metabolic Research Ward of a university hospital during the early 1950's. This hospital is much like our University Hospital and Research Center. Most of the patients on the ward were suffering from diseases for which there were no known cures. The doctors were seeking both to provide therapy for their patients and to find out more about these diseases.

> The fact that the hormones with which the Metabolic group was experimenting had unanticipated negative side effects on patients and that they were proving to be ameliorative rather than curative, along with their difficulties in keeping alive and managing the clinical course of patients who had undergone experimental surgery, account for many of the stressful problems which these research physicians had at the time this study was made.[19]

Fox reports on the investigators' constant concern with justifying the risks which they were asking their subjects to accept, with the quality of care which was provided for the patients, and with providing them with enough information so that they could give their "voluntary consent" to research. In a published research report the investigators from the Metabolic Group made explicit their concern with balancing risk against benefit:

> Were such procedures "justified as an experimental approach in man"? Could they be "carried out with reasonable safety" in patients? . . . What therapeutic benefits, if any, could be derived from these procedures?[20]

---

[19] Fox, *Experiment Perilous*, p. 19.

[20] George W. Thorn, J. Hartwell Harrison, John P. Merrill, Modestino G. Criscitiello, Thomas F. Frawley, and John T. Finkenstaedt, "Clinical Studies on Bilateral Complete Adrenalectomy in Patients with Severe Hypertensive Vascular Disease," *Annals of Internal Medicine*, 37, no. 5 (November, 1952): 972–1005, cited in Fox, *Experiment Perilous*, p. 33.

In accordance with the Nuremberg Code, not only were the risks of the proposed research evaluated against benefits, but oral and sometimes written consent was obtained from all patients.[21] The Metabolic Group was a small research group in intensive interaction both among themselves and with their patient-subjects, and highly concerned with the ethics of research. In such a situation—which is actually far from universal in medical research —any researcher would have to become aware of the ethical problems of research.

The group research situation which Stewart Perry describes in *The Human Nature of Science* provides an interesting contrast. Fox's Metabolic Group was well-established, with formal procedures for dealing with consent, and had considerable practice in evaluating research against therapy; new members could be socialized effectively by the group. In the case which Perry describes, a new research institute had been established, and a new staff, some of whom had not been engaged in research before, was attempting to establish guidelines for a psychiatric research program.[22]

In discussions over the two years covered by Perry's observations, the staff indicated its dissatisfaction with attempts to solve the dilemma of research versus therapy. They were agreed that therapy was to come first and that research must not interfere in any way with the patient's progress: a straightforward principle, but one difficult to apply in practice. There were no clear, established therapeutic procedures for dealing with the patients' problems, and the investigators were not certain of how to combine the roles of therapist and investigator—or if indeed they could be combined at all.

One research project, which Perry calls the First LSD Project, was the subject of much discussion. The question as the investigators defined it, and as Perry emphasizes, was whether subjects who refused to submit to research procedures could be discharged from the research unit, that is, denied therapy. One subject of two chosen for the research refused all cooperation; the other withdrew consent after the first of several planned administrations of an experimental drug with unpleasant effects. Although the second subject later agreed to the procedure, it was never carried out. The research project was never formally abandoned, but it was never completed.

It is of special interest that, according to Perry, the decision not to continue the research was not based on the same clear standards for human experimentation used by the Metabolic Research Group.

> The LSD project revisions involved the invocation of a moral basis for action, for the scientist as a clinical researcher does not discard his allegiance to the basic moral commitments of his culture. . . . When the conferees asked them-

---

[21] Fox, *Experiment Perilous*, p. 112.

[22] Stewart Perry, *The Human Nature of Science* (New York: The Free Press, 1966).

selves whether they were "unfriendly" or not, *they were harking back to broader and more fundamental standards for judgment than those explicit in the medical subculture.* They were in fact not only wondering if they were being good doctors, they were asking themselves if they were good people.[23]

It is true that the ethical norms that define appropriate behavior for the researcher vis-à-vis his subjects are not scientific norms, but the "basic moral commitments" of the researchers' culture are not adequate to insure the protection of research subjects' rights and welfare and at the same time promote needed research. Some of the investigators' difficulty in resolving the dilemma of science and therapy might have been resolved if there had been any explicit and prior consideration of the right of the research subject to give his informed consent to any procedure. The discussion of the LSD Project was precipitated by a subject's refusal to repeat an experience, the administration of a drug, which had been frightening and which she had not been told about before agreeing to enter the research institute as a patient-subject. Only after this point was any full disclosure of the research protocol made to the subjects, *in order to obtain their cooperation*, not to comply with their rights as research subjects.

It might seem from these two case studies of ongoing research that physician-investigators could not, in fact, avoid an awareness of the ethical issues in biomedical research. Both Fox and Perry assert the pervasiveness of the dilemma of science and therapy and the resulting stresses for the researcher. Both also emphasize the active cooperation of the subject in the research process, the relationship which develops between the investigator and his subjects. In the case reported by Fox, procedures are serious, have significant risk; in the case reported by Perry, the procedures are unpleasant, even painful, without offering any therapeutic benefit. The relationship with the patients in both cases continued over a long period of time and the subjects' cooperation was essential. There were few patients and the researchers were acting as therapists as well as investigators.

Our own data indicate that these circumstances—research in which there is serious risk or in which the researcher has a continuing relationship with his subjects—are in fact just those in which there is most stress for the researcher. Respondents were asked: "Have you ever found yourself becoming involved emotionally with the people serving as subjects in your research to an extent greater than you deem desirable for a researcher?" Fifty-six respondents (17%) said that they had become so involved with their subjects; this had happened, they said, when they were working with subjects who were seriously ill and could not be helped, when research procedures seemed to involve risk which was not balanced by benefits for the subjects,

---

[23] *Ibid.*, p. 99 (Emphasis supplied).

or when they got to know their subjects well and became more concerned with them as persons than as subjects. We also have some data on how prevalent these stress-producing conditions are. First, only 17% of our respondents reported ever becoming excessively involved with their subjects. Second, the majority of the projects reported by our respondents did not involve such stress; 44% of the 422 research projects mentioned involved no risk for the subjects, and another 45% involved only very little risk. It is not risk alone, of course, which creates ethical problems, but risk in relation to the benefits for the subjects; in 18% of the research projects the risk was judged to be relatively high in proportion to the benefits for the subjects (less favorable studies) and in 8% of them the risk was judged to be relatively high in proportion to benefits for the subjects, for others, and for the advance of medical science (least favorable studies). Seven projects involved at least relatively large, significant risk to the subjects without equivalent benefits.[24]

In most research projects, then, the investigator is not faced with a decision about serious, life-threatening procedures for his patient-subjects. Third, there is some evidence, although we did not collect it systematically, that there are mechanisms which protect investigators from emotional involvement in research by limiting their contact with their subjects. We have already noted that in many cases patients are identified and research procedures carried out by interns and residents. Using interns and residents to handle patient contact would reduce strain for the investigators; and the interns and residents could accept the ethical decisions affecting their patients as made by other, more knowledgeable physicians, thereby reducing any strain they themselves might feel. Much research is brief, involving simple measurements on large numbers of subjects. Much research could be, and some is, conducted without the knowledge and cooperation of the subjects. The patients' involvement is not necessarily conscious, long-term, or painful.

The research group and the institution in which research is carried out, then, may be important in socializing those researchers who have not become aware of the ethics of human experimentation before they began their actual research. However, it has its limitations as a socializing process. We have seen that only a minority of research projects have the characteristics of risk and patient contact which seem to make researchers aware of research ethics. Further, only 5% of our researcher respondents reported their colleagues in research as influencing their awareness of research ethics and 3% reported increased awareness from the formal regulations of the institution governing the use of human subjects. When we compare these

---

[24] For descriptions of six of these least justifiable studies and the researchers who engaged in them see Chapter 8.

indicators of the influence of the research group and institution with the 8% whose awareness resulted from the negative reactions of their own or others' subjects we may conclude that there is a need for formal socialization into research ethics in the research setting, a need which is not being met at the present time.

THE CONSEQUENCES OF ETHICAL SOCIALIZATION FOR EXPRESSED STANDARDS AND BEHAVIOR

Up to this point in this chapter, we have been concerned simply with *describing* the processes through which biomedical researchers are socialized into a concern for the rights and welfare of research subjects as our own respondents, and a few other observers, have perceived them. We come, finally, to the problem of the consequences of these processes of ethical socialization for ethical standards and practices. Since the medical school is the locus of most of the ethical socialization that does occur and because it should presumably be one of the most important structures for such socialization, we shall look first at our data on the effects of medical school socialization. How effective, then, is the ethical socialization which, as we have seen, only a minority of students receive in medical school? We expected, of course, that those reporting such experiences would be less permissive in their willingness to subject human subjects to risk and more alert to the moral desirability of obtaining informed consent from those who were asked to undergo experimental procedures. But our expectation was realized only in small measure and in certain qualified ways.

So far as expressed standards on the two issues of consent and risk are concerned, for example, those researchers who reported *any* ethical training during the course of medical school training—classes, or seminars devoted to ethical issues, or awareness through practice procedures or work on experimental animals, or discussions with teachers or fellow students—were only slightly less permissive on the bone metabolism study, which involved the risk-benefit issue, than their colleagues who reported no such experiences. That is, there was a smaller proportion of the former who would permit the risks of the bone metabolism study to be done at all. And on the pulmonary function study, where the issue is that of informed consent, socialization seems to have had practically no effect on expressed standards. It is only a small and approximately equal minority of those ethically socialized in medical school and those not so socialized that shows itself sensitive to the consent issue.

In order to see if there was a cumulative effect of *multiple* socialization experiences in medical school, and to increase the number of cases for analysis, we compared those respondents who reported no experiences at all with those reporting one, or two, or three. Even in this situation of possibly cumulative effects, there is no significant difference among the four groups in the recognition of the desirability of *informed consent*, as measured by their responses to the pulmonary function study.[25] But there are some interesting differences among the groups on the bone metabolism study, where *risk-benefit* is at issue. As Table 6.8 shows, those reporting socialization experi-

Table 6.8. Percentage of Respondents Reporting Formal Socialization Experiences during Medical School by Willingness to Permit Study of Bone Metabolism

Reaction to Proposed Study	Number of Formal Experiences			
	None	One	Two or Three	Total
Relatively permissive	30%	13%	11%	20%
Moderate	17	30	28	24
Strict	53	57	61	56
Totals	100% (112)	100% (91)	100% (53)	100% (256)
	44%	36%	21%	100%

ences in medical school were less permissive on this issue. Thirty per cent of the respondents who reported no socialization experiences would have permitted the dangerous radioactive treatment in the study of bone metabolism in children if there were only a 10–30% chance of an important discovery; but only 13% of those reporting one experience and 11% of those reporting two or three.

At the same time that socialization into research ethics in medical schools is apparently only minimally effective, there does seem to be a kind of socialization going on during medical school and later, a socialization into the positive value of research science, which does lead to more permissive standards on the consent and risk-benefit issues. It will be remembered that the very first question on socialization that we asked our respondents was, "Can you remember when you first became aware of the issues involved in the use of human subjects in research?" We have already presented the results of the response to this question. In addition, as further parts of this question, we asked two other questions, "Under what circumstances

---

[25] Note Dr. Jay Katz' remark, in response to those who speak of the importance of the competent investigator as a guarantee of concern with the issue of informed consent: "If disclosure and consent are posited as important problems for medical research, these commentators forgot to realize that physicians could not draw on systematic prior training." Katz, "The Education of the Physician-Investigator," p. 487.

did you first become aware?" and "Do you remember your reaction?" In telling us about these circumstances and about their reactions, our respondents mentioned, as we had hoped they would, a variety of experiences which referred not only to the information conveyed by those experiences but also to some *emotional or moral reaction* they had had to them.

We grouped these responses into two categories. The first we called the "negative reaction" category. In this category we put respondents who told us how they became aware of research which endangered or harmed some subjects, or which was done without the subjects' knowledge or consent, or which was unnecessary or poorly designed. In these responses, the respondent seemed to feel that the rights and welfare of the subjects, which ought to have been the primary consideration, had been neglected in favor of research. They seemed to be preferring humane therapy to science.

The second category we called the "value of research" category. In this case the respondent told us how, as a student, he had learned to admire heroic researchers; or how, in his own research, he had seen the necessity of going beyond animal experimentation to the use of humans; or, again, how his early contacts with patients had shown him the need for new scientific knowledge. The preference for these respondents seemed to be on the needs of science. These may be the people to whom Henry Beecher is referring when he says:

> Nowadays, we have a new generation of physicians whose primary interests are scientific: this is good only as long as the scientist proceeds and coordinates his activities with those of the patient's physician; only then will any "too casual" view of the patient as subject be avoided.[26]

These two categories of reaction, these two orientations to biomedical research, the one negative and emphasizing the protection of the subject's rights and welfare and the other positive and emphasizing the importance of scientific investigation, seem to represent distinctive outcomes of the total ethical socialization process for our respondents. The two categories manifest what we have called the dilemma of science and therapy and they have consequences, as we shall now see, for the conduct of experimentation using human subjects.

Table 6.9 tells one part of the story about the consequences of these different types of reactions. In regard to the risk issue as measured by response to the bone metabolism study, for example, only 17% of those with a negative reaction to research as against 40% of those with a positive reaction were permissive. (It should be noted that, to maintain firm standards on who was to be classified positive, who negative, we placed many respond-

---

[26] Henry K. Beecher, *Research and the Individual*, p. 42.

Table 6.9. Respondents' Reactions to First Awareness of the Ethical Issues of Human Experimentation by Willingness to Permit Study of Bone Metabolism

Reaction to Proposed Study	Reaction to First Awareness			Total
	Negative	*Neutral*	*Positive*	*Total*
Relatively permissive	17%	17%	40%	19%
Moderate	29	25	24	26
Strict	54	58	36	55
	100% (83)	100% (166)	100% (25)	100% (274)

ents in a neutral category and have included them in this table.) And correlatively, the table shows, more of the negative than the positive respondents are strict in their judgments about the risks involved in the bone metabolism study. The same situation holds with regard to the informed consent issue as measured by the pulmonary function study; type of reaction has consequences. Some 29% of those in the negative reaction category (87 all together) volunteered, without further probing by our interviewers, that they would not approve the study as presented unless the issue of consent was properly taken care of in the protocol, whereas only 8% of those in the positive reaction category (26 all together) were similarly alert to the consent issue. In sum, we find that those who reacted to their first awareness of the ethical issues of human experimentation with an increased concern for the importance of scientific discovery, rather than a concern for the patient's welfare, are more willing to accept risk and are less alert to the requirement of informed consent than those whose first reaction was negative. And it is clear, as a matter of general interest, that it is not so much that professional socialization, even by itself, cannot be effective, but that it may be of the wrong kind for certain purposes, or it may be given in the wrong proportions, or it may have unintended effects.

Up to this point in our discussion of the effects of socialization, the careful reader may have noted, we have been speaking only of effects on expressed standards with regard to the consent and risk-benefit issues. Such effects could occur, also, of course, for actual behavior, as measured by the reports the researchers gave us about their own behavior on their studies. However, we have found that using the third unit of analysis (the role unit) as we did in Chapters 4 and 5, there are no clear and direct relationships between socialization experiences alone and reported behavior. Still, it will be remembered from an earlier statement in this chapter that it is our theoretical position that socialization, as one of a set of variables in a social system, is partly independent, partly interdependent with the other variables, in producing its effects. In the next chapter, therefore, we shall show how socialization, in interdependence with a number of structural conditions—collaboration-group structure, patterns of authority, and informal interaction structures, all of which would probably be defined by Freidson and Carlin as "work-context"—does produce effects on behavior. In the next chapter, after describing some of our findings about these structural conditions in which our researchers work, we will examine the interdependence between such socialization variables as number of socializing experiences in medical school and type of reaction to first ethical awareness, on the one hand, and such structural variables as organization of the collaboration group and patterns of authority among researchers, on the other.

7

SOCIAL CONTROL: SOME PATTERNS AND CONSEQUENCES OF COLLABORATION GROUPS AND INFORMAL INTERACTION STRUCTURES

The second type of social control we have studied consists of those structures and processes that bring the pressures of informal social interaction to bear on behalf of conformity or deviance. In this chapter, therefore, we inquire how scientific collaboration groups and other informal interaction structures may affect the "strict" and "permissive" patterns we have discerned among biomedical researchers. Here again we shall proceed by first reporting the methods and instruments we used to collect our data in this area. Then we shall suggest some of the ways that informal structures, just by themselves, *may* influence expressed standards and actual behavior in the use of human subjects. Finally, we shall suggest certain effects that informal interaction structures, in interaction with certain socialization patterns, may have on actual behavior as reported to us by our respondents. Informal colleague interaction, through the processes of collaboration, ethical consultation, and decision-making, has possible and actual effects on standards and behavior which we shall now seek to describe.

DATA AND METHODS

Our data on collaboration groups and informal interaction structures were collected by personal interview in our Intensive Two-Institution Study (Chapter 2). By asking a series of sociometric questions of our respondents, we hoped to identify significant members of specific sectors of their work and informal interaction environments. We hoped, that is, to identify those researchers or other colleagues who, for each respondent, were in positions where they could, if the overt need arose, or would be likely to, in a more latent and continuous way, exercise some control over his standards and behavior. We asked, first, for the names of all colleagues with rank of resident or higher with whom our interviewees collaborated on each of their research studies (up to a total of eight) where human subjects were used. Collaborators thus named were recorded in such a way that the names for each study were kept separate if the interviewee was engaged in more than one project.

Respondents were then asked if any of the collaborators they had named, if they had named one or more, would not co-author scientific papers resulting from the study. We were attempting here to differentiate between higher and lower status members of collaboration groupings. In addition, each respondent was asked: "Is any of those you have named, including yourself, the leader of the research group(s), or do you consider your research group(s) to be a collaboration of equals?"

Any researchers named by an interviewee as collaborators who were not already on our list to be contacted for an interview were then placed on the list and contacted. By using this technique, called snowball sampling, we hoped to be able to interview all members of a fairly large number of collaboration groups. We assumed that collaborators would exert a controlling influence on each other depending upon the nature of their internalized ethical standards. We looked to the members of collaboration groups, if there were any, as sources of mutual social control.

When each of an interviewee's sociometric choices as collaborators for a given study were interviewed and when at least 80% of all collaborators that were mentioned by *any* of the members of the group were interviewed, the interviewee in question was assigned a whole series of attributes of his collaborators as "contextual"[1] characteristics. For example, if at least 75% of our interviewees' sociometric choices for a given study on a given dimension were homogeneous, their choices were classified as *homogeneous* on that dimension. In all other cases, they were classified as *mixed*. The same was done for all collaborators interviewed, regardless of whether each was chosen by that interviewee. In this or in a similar way a large number of contextual attributes were coded, including such things as political views, average number of citations, average number of publications in the last five years, and ethical standards as measured by the mean response of the group to the hypothetical proposals.

An interviewee's sociometric choices were given the special attention outlined above because we felt that they might represent the collaboration group as he saw it. In other words, the choices might be more likely than those who were not chosen to be the group members who would exert social control on the researcher in question. All contextual attributes were coded in these two ways.

---

[1] For a discussion of "contextual" attributes of the individual, see Paul F. Lazarsfeld and Herbert Menzel, "On the Relation Between Individual and Collective Properties," in *Complex Organizations: A Sociological Reader*, Amitai Etzioni, ed. (New York: Holt, Rinehart and Winston, 1961), pp. 422–440.

In addition, if the study was a collaborative one and if the principal investigator was interviewed, each member of the group who was interviewed and who acknowledged his participation in the study (once again a requirement in order to be a unit of analysis) was given attributes of the principal investigator as contextual attributes. If the interviewee was himself the principal investigator, that was his attribute. All other collaborators in the group were then given as attributes the principal investigator's ethical standards as indicated by his response to the hypothetical bone metabolism study. The purpose of all this was to lay out as fully as possible for each interviewee who was in one or more collaborative studies the relevant characteristics of the researchers with whom he collaborated and to record their status in the collaboration group.

Interviewees were also asked for the number of interns, medical students, and graduate students participating with them in each study. These data were not coded, but it is clear from an inspection of the questionnaires that participation by people of those types in studies involving human subjects were strikingly small in the two institutions we studied. To become a researcher, or at least an acknowledged one, who uses human subjects one must apparently be at least a resident or the equivalent.

We also asked respondents for the names of other researchers in the institution who were not collaborators on the project in question, with whom they had had discussions resulting in an exchange of ideas or in picking up needed information. The frequency of these contacts was coded, but the attributes of the specific researchers were not. Not enough of them were interviewed since we only snowballed for additional collaborators. The same is true for our sociometric data on therapeutic consulting relationships.[2]

In order to identify the people with whom our interviewees discussed ethical questions if and when they arose, we asked the following question:

> Sometimes conducting research on humans can confront an investigator with serious ethical dilemmas, the solutions to which are not always clear. During the past year, how many times have you discussed with one of your colleagues in this institution the ethical issues involved in the utilization of human subjects or an ethical dilemma present in your own research?
>
> A. In general terms, not connected with your own research?
>
> _____ times
>
> A.1. *IF AT ALL:* With whom have you discussed these issues?
>
> B. As they may have arisen in your own research?
>
> _____ times
>
> B.1. *IF AT ALL:* With whom have you discussed these issues?

Because of the centrality of this question for our goal of identifying possible

---

[2] See questions 6 and 7 of the interview schedule, reproduced in Appendix II.

agents of social control for a particular interviewee, both the frequency of these discussions and some of the characteristics of the individuals who were mentioned were coded. In particular, the mean ethical standards of those involved with the interviewee in such discussions were coded when the persons mentioned had been interviewed. Again, because of lack of time and resources, we did not snowball when persons were mentioned in these questions who were not already on our list to be contacted.

The names of luncheon associates and colleagues whom an interviewee saw socially within the past year were also solicited, along with the frequency of such contacts. The frequency of these contacts was coded but, again, no contextual attributes were assigned on the basis of particular names mentioned.

Finally, in our search for sociometric data that might help us to analyze the informal social control mechanisms that influenced ethical standards and behavior, each interviewee was asked to name the three physicians, whether in his institution or not, with whom he was most friendly. The mean response to the hypothetical research proposals of any friends interviewed was coded as an attribute of the interviewee.

Because we did not snowball our population on any dimension except that of collaboration, the number of interviewees who could be given, as contextual attributes, the characteristics of their choices on other items was fairly small. In addition, the reliability of contextual attributes that are based on small proportions of the number of choices actually made by an interviewee, as in the case of all contextual attributes except those based on collaboration choices, is necessarily much less than it would have been if we had snowballed along additional dimensions. In the case of collaborators' attributes, as mentioned above, we only coded when at least 80% of the collaborators had been interviewed.

In summary, we have tried to identify potential agents of informal social control in the immediate social environment of our biomedical researchers and to measure the likelihood that they will facilitate or hinder a researcher who would engage in a study with risks in excess of the benefits for the human subjects involved. As the analysis to follow will show we have had mixed results in our attempt to understand the workings of informal social control by proceeding in this way, but we have isolated some interesting findings.

SOME PATTERNS AND CONSEQUENCES OF INFORMAL INTERACTION

First, let us see how many of the 424 human studies on which we have data are collaborative as opposed to being done by one man. As Table 7.1

Table 7.1. Number of Investigators for Each Study

One-man study	19%
Two	27
Three	24
Four or more	30
	100% (424)

shows, modern biomedical research on humans is highly collaborative; only 19% of the studies on which we gathered data had only one investigator. Though the data are not exactly comparable, Hagstrom's figures on collaboration and teamwork in three experimental disciplines at the University of California are of the same general order of magnitude.[3] And Zuckerman reports that at least 40% of scientific papers in the biological sciences are multi-authored.[4]

It is worthy of mention, though the differences are slight, that researchers working alone less often engage in less favorable studies for subjects than do researchers in pairs or groups of three or more. It may be that researchers planning to do a study with risks in excess of the therapeutic benefits need some social support; they feel more vulnerable by themselves. Or, it could be that in order to use procedures which involve significant risks, except in the case of administering drugs, more than one researcher is required. Inspection of the interview schedules shows that studies involving some risk, moderate risk or high risk for the subjects most often involve drug tests, catheterizations, and biopsies. Usually the last two types of procedures would tend to require more than one person. Table 7.2 shows this slight relationship. In the next chapter some of the seven studies least favorable of all for the subjects will be singled out for intensive analysis. It should be noted here that none of them involves just one investigator; all are collaborative studies.

Since 81% of the human studies on which we have data are collaborative, it is important that we look closely at the kinds of researchers who choose to work together. Do the social selection mechanisms which operate to bring researchers together operate randomly with respect to those individual characteristics that are related to ethical standards and practices? Or,

---

[3] Hagstrom, *op. cit.*, p. 128. At the University of California scientists in three disciplines work alone in the following proportions: physics 3% (30); chemistry 12% (26); experimental biology 38% (24).

[4] Harriet Zuckerman, "Patterns of Name Ordering Among Authors of Scientific Papers: A Study of Social Symbolism and Its Ambiguity," *American Journal of Sociology*, 74, no. 3 (1968): 277.

Table 7.2. Per Cent Engaged in Less Favorable Studies by Number of Collaborators, Using Mean Estimate of All Collaborators Interviewed

	Number of Collaborators			
	One	*Two*	*Three*	*Four or More*
Per cent engaged in less favorable studies	14% (62)	19% (103)	19% (91)	24% (119)

do researchers of like backgrounds and ethical standards collaborate with each other?

Important ethical decisions for a study involving human subjects are made by the researcher(s) involved at two significant points in time: when the study is designed and during its progress. When the study is designed, important decisions such as the following need to be made: (1) the procedures to be used to gather the data; (2) the population from which subjects will be selected; and (3) the kind of consent to be obtained, if any. There may be other important decisions to be made, but let us look at these more closely as illustrative types.

The data-gathering procedures selected by the researchers during the design phase largely determine the amount of risk and discomfort subjects will undergo. To the extent that procedures are available which would produce roughly comparable data, but which vary in the risk and discomfort involved, important ethical choices have to be made. It may be that only one procedure is presently known that would produce the necessary data. In that case the decision is whether or not to do the study at all.

The decision on the population from which to select subjects also often takes place during the design phase. Who will be exposed to the risk and discomfort, if any, and who will benefit, if anyone? Are normal controls necessary, for whom there will certainly be no benefit? Should private patients be used if possible, or should ward patients be used?

Third, decisions are made about how particular people will be recruited as subjects. Is it necessary to obtain the consent of potential subjects? If so, how detailed should the explanation be? These are all ethical decisions which are generally made before the study is begun, and potential collaborators who may be approached by a principal investigator who has designed a study make an ethical decision when they choose or choose not to participate. Long-term collaborators who design studies together, of course, are involved in the ethical decisions right from the start.

Many types of ethical decisions, however, also have to be made while the study is in progress. Should a subject who is reacting adversely to an experimental drug be dropped from the study? One of the case studies in the next chapter illustrates this ethical dilemma and the resultant conflict among the collaborators over how the dilemma should be resolved. Should the research design be modified or altered during the study in order to take advantage of fortuitous circumstances? When decisions of these kinds are made during the design or progress of a study, one collaborator may certainly influence the thoughts and actions of another. Here, the implications of the social selection process are great. If researchers who have the same general ethical perspectives tend to collaborate with one another, the ethical decisions proposed by one collaborator will less frequently be questioned by the others.

The kinds of decisions during the actual course of a study on which intercollaborator influences most frequently have an effect were not measured by us systematically and at different points in the research process. In another study, it would be desirable to do just that. We do have data, however, on the ethical standards and other characteristics of researchers who collaborate, and on the criteria researchers say they would use in choosing a collaborator for a study involving human subjects. We can say something, then, about what affects the first decision stage.

Looking first at the criteria researchers say they use in choosing collaborators, we asked the following question: "What three characteristics do you most want to know about another researcher before entering into a collaborative relationship with him?" Table 7.3 shows the proportion of

Table 7.3. Proportion of Researchers Mentioning Each Characteristic Desirable in a Collaborator

Scientific ability	86%
Motivation to work hard	45%
Personality	43%
Intellectual honesty	32%
Practical skills or financial resources	9%
Same orientation toward science	7%
Scientific prestige	6%
Ethical concern for research subjects	6%

interviewees who mentioned each characteristic. The answers to this question were not precoded and, therefore, the characteristics shown in the table were developed during the coding process. Also, this question was not included in the shortened mailed questionnaire that was returned by 35 researchers, so the base here is 352 interviews. All of the general characteristics listed seem self-explanatory except for "intellectual honesty." Coded in that category are two general kinds of statements: (1) the potential collaborator must be a person who does not distort data to fit his conceptions; and (2) the potential collaborator must be fair in dividing up credit for work done and must not steal the ideas of other collaborators for his own use.

As Table 7.3 makes clear, our respondents rarely (6%) said that a researcher's ethical standards were relevant in choosing him as a collaborator. The two most frequently mentioned characteristics, ability and motivation, are related directly to the scientific work to be done. Here again, the greater salience of "value of research" over "humane therapy" seems to show itself. The high number of times personality is mentioned is not unexpected given the frequently great intensity and longevity of interaction required to complete a piece of research.

According to our interviewees, then, ethical standards are not a highly salient consideration when compared to other factors as criteria for selecting collaborators.[5] When we examine our other data, however, we find a consistent latent tendency for our researchers to be collaborating with researchers who do in fact share their ethical standards. In Table 7.4, for each interviewee who is in a collaborative study we have crosstabulated his response to the bone metabolism hypothetical research proposal, first, with the mean response of only his sociometric choices and, then, with the mean of the group as a whole, that is, using all his collaborators interviewed. In order to be included in the table in which the standards of only his sociometric choices are presented, all of a researcher's choices had to have been interviewed. In the case of the table in which the whole group's standards are presented, at least 80% of the other members of the group, not including the researcher in question, had to have been interviewed. In neither mean is the response to the hypothetical question of the researcher who forms the unit of analysis included. It is always the mean of his collaborators' expressed ethical standards. Interviewees were classified as permissive in their response

---

[5] After reading, in a brief summary of our research sent to all our respondents, about this finding of the relative lack of salience of ethical concern as against scientific ability in the set of characteristics mentioned as desirable in collaborators, one respondent wrote to protest this finding, saying: "Since you merely asked people to list '*a set*' of valuable characteristics extemporaneously, one would *naturally* [emphasis added] first think of scientific ability, hard work, etc." But, to the sociologist, there is nothing more "natural" about a greater salience for scientific ability than for ethical concern. It is the sociologist's task to find the conditions under which one characteristic is more salient, or more anything else, than another. This is our task in this book: to explain why, with the present dilemma of science and therapy, somewhat more salience is being given to science than to ethical concern for subjects.

The greater salience of science does not mean, of course, that there is no concern at all for humane and ethical treatment of subjects. But the relative salience of values has effects on behavior, and this is what we are concerned with in the finding which our respondent has protested.

Table 7.4. Permissiveness of Expressed Ethical Standards of Individual by Permissiveness of Expressed Ethical Standards of His Collaborators

Permissiveness of Individual's Socio-metric Choices	Permissiveness of Individual			
	Permissive	Moderate	Strict	Total
Permissive	38%	51%	27%	36%
Moderate	25	15	19	19
Strict	37	34	54	45
Totals	100% (51)	100% (77)	100% (140)	100% (268)
	19%	29%	52%	100%

Permissiveness of All Individual's Collaborators				
Permissive	32%	46%	18%	28%
Moderate	35	15	31	27
Strict	33	39	51	45
Totals	100% (51)	100% (72)	100% (144)	100% (267)
	19%	27%	54%	100%

to the bone metabolism hypothetical proposal if they would approve the study under the condition that the chance of an important discovery was 30% or less. Strict interviewees would not approve the study regardless of the probability of success, and moderates are any who fall between those extremes.[6] Though the percentages are not ordinal but curvilinear in the top row of both tables, and though moderate researchers are least likely to collaborate with other moderate researchers, the overall tendency is for researchers with approximately the same expressed ethical standards, as measured by their responses to our bone metabolism hypothetical research proposal, to collaborate with each other more frequently than with researchers holding different standards.

It will be remembered that a second hypothetical research proposal, involving a pulmonary function study in which consent was the issue, was also presented to our interviewees for review. Though the data will not be presented here, when responses to that proposal are analyzed in the same way as those to the first proposal, the differences are similar but smaller. Researchers who are sensitive to consent as an ethical issue tend to collabo-

---

[6] The cutting points for the mean response of sociometric choices and all collaborators were the same, except that means of 5.1 to 6.0 were called strict. On the interview schedule the choices were numbered 1–6 with 6 being strictest category.

rate with others who share that sensitivity. There is, in addition, some tendency for collaboration groups to be homogeneous religiously and politically, though the differences are not large. We will concentrate here, therefore, on the implications for social control of homogeneity in expressed ethical standards.

In sum, though our interviewees did not indicate that ethical standards are a conscious criterion for selecting their collaborators, in fact they do tend to select collaborators who have the same ethical standards as they do. This tendency to similarity in expressed standards, as we indicated earlier, tends to decrease the likelihood that one collaborator will disagree with ethical decisions made by another. That is fine where both collaborators have strict standards. But where collaborators tend to share permissive standards, they are not likely to enforce the stricter ethical norms of the majority of the wider research community on each other.

It will be recalled that we also asked our respondents to whom they went in the past year to discuss ethical questions arising in their own research. Since those named were very frequently not researchers themselves or, if researchers, were not interviewed, in the case of only 122 interviewees could we classify the ethical standards of those with whom they discuss ethical problems in their research. The data here are slightly encouraging from the point of view of social control, for they indicate a tendency for investigators to discuss their ethical dilemmas with other researchers who have different ethical standards from those they themselves have. Some researchers may be trying to insure that they are neither too strict (not so good a process?) nor too permissive (a better one?). The differences are not large, however, and the total sample size, remember, is small, as is shown in Table 7.5.

Thus, though our data on these matters are by no means conclusive, informal intercolleague influence seems to be organized around two different social selection processes. Researchers tend to choose collaborators who share the same ethical standards as they do, but sometimes they may also counteract this reinforcing influence by discussing ethical dilemmas they have in their research with researchers who hold to different standards.

Are permissive individuals and permissive collaboration groups more likely to be engaged in less favorable studies for the subjects, however? Our data indicate that the answer is "no" for the more innocuous studies where risks are only slightly in excess of benefits. But, as we shall see in some of the cases presented in the next chapter, when six of the seven studies with the least favorable of all risks-benefits ratios are analyzed, the opposite trend is clearly evident. Many studies where the risks are just slightly in excess of the benefits for the subjects (the majority of the "less favorable" studies) are apparently within a "zone of indifference" for many otherwise strict re-

Table 7.5. Permissiveness of Expressed Ethical Standards of Individual by Mean Permissiveness of Expressed Ethical Standards of Persons with Whom He Discusses Ethical Dilemmas in His Own Research

Permissiveness of Individual's Ethical Counselors	Permissiveness of Individual			
	Permissive	Moderate	Strict	Total
Permissive	19%	35%	30%	29%
Moderate	14	18	21	19
Strict	67	47	49	52
Totals	100% (21)	100% (34)	100% (67)	100% (122)
	17%	28%	55%	100%

searchers. In order for a more problematic study to be done, however, the principal investigator must, the data in the next chapter suggest, have either very permissive ethical standards and/or be subject to the structured pressures, documented in Chapters 4 and 5, coming from the competitive structures of science as a whole and of the local research institution.

ETHICAL CONSEQUENCES OF THE INTERACTION OF INFORMAL INTERACTION AND SOCIALIZATION STRUCTURES

In the attempt to discover some of the sources of conforming and deviant behavior involving informal interaction structures, we decided to consider certain multivariate possibilities. For example, we decided to see if the combination of certain informal interaction structures with certain socialization structures and processes might not be among the determinants we were seeking to find. As the following results indicate, we had some success with this multivariate strategy.

As one part of our analysis of collaboration groups, we drew sociograms for each study, using the responses to our questions about who were members of the collaboration group, who was in charge, and who might or might not get authorship. The responses showed a certain amount of disagreement on these matters, even as to membership itself. Apparently, in the busy, multiverse, and endlessly beginning-and-ending world of biomedical research collaboration groups, the structure and even membership of particular groups is not always entirely clear. Because of this obscurity, as a rough indicator of position in the group we used the number of times an investigator was actually named as a member of a group divided by the number of possible times he could have been so named. Those investigators who received 75% or more of the possible choices in their collaboration groups are called "highly chosen" members; others are the "less chosen." Furthermore, we assumed that those who were highly chosen were so because they were highly visible to the other members of the group as active in the planning and direction of the research. We also assumed that this significant activity in the group gave them some degree of relatively greater effectiveness in making those decisions about the research design and the choice of subjects which had ethical implications. Such greater effectiveness, we assumed finally, would make it more possible to act in accord with one's socialization experiences. Those with more medical school experiences would be less likely than those with no medical school socialization to be engaged in less favorable studies if they worked alone or if they were highly chosen. Those who were less chosen would not be able to act on their predispositions, and the number of medical school socialization experiences which they reported would not be related to their behavior. As Table 7.6 shows,

Table 7.6.   Per Cent Engaged in Less Favorable Studies by Number of Experiences in Medical School and Position in Research Group

Position in Research Group	Number of Experiences in Medical School		
	None	*One*	*Two or Three*
Works alone	14% (97)	13% (80)	8% (61)
Highly chosen	32% (90)	22% (67)	21% (34)
Less chosen	10% (42)	13% (31)	11% (18)

this seems to be what we find, although the differences are not large.

Those whose reaction to their first awareness of the problems of biomedical research was a "negative reaction" (indicating the value of humane therapy) would be less likely to engage in unfavorable studies than those whose reaction was a "positive" one (indicating the value of research) if they worked alone or were highly chosen. Those who were less chosen would be unable to act on their predispositions and we would expect no relationship between their reaction to the ethical problems of research and their present behavior. Again, as we see in Table 7.7, the data do not contradict such an explanation, although the small number of cases in some cells makes an adequate test impossible.

As a result of this finding that position in the informal interaction structure seems to interact with socialization experiences to affect conforming and deviant behavior in the use of human subjects, we wondered if other structural conditions, even more formal ones, might not have the same interactive effect. For example, we wondered if the structural position of rank in the local institution might not have this effect. Since the researchers with

Table 7.7.   Per Cent Engaged in Less Favorable Studies by Reaction to First Awareness of Ethical Issues and Position in Research Group

Position in Research Group	Reaction to First Awareness of Ethical Issues		
	Negative	*Neutral*	*Positive*
Works alone	10% (67)	13% (148)	18% (34)
Highly chosen	28% (65)	26% (133)	40% (15)
Less chosen	23% (31)	13% (69)	— (9)

higher rank have more authority, more control of resources, and more prestige, we expected that they would be more free than those of lower rank to select problems, colleagues, and subject populations in accordance with ethical standards established by their previous socialization experiences. As we saw when we reviewed Stephen Miller's description of the exchange pattern at the Harvard Medical Unit at Boston City Hospital, a pattern in which the interns exchange information about patients who might be subjects for researchers in return for teaching by and consultation with those researchers, the question was not whether the proposed research procedures were ethical or not, but whether the interns and residents were free to act in accordance with their own ethical standards. Local rank has its effects at the B.C.H. and so it does, as Tables 7.8 and 7.9 show, in the two hospital and re-

Table 7.8.   Per Cent Engaged in Less Favorable Studies by Number of Experiences in Medical School and Rank in Local Institution

Rank in Local Institution	Number of Experiences		
	None	*One*	*Two or Three*
Associate attending or Attending	26% (110)	12% (65)	9% (47)
Assistant attending	11% (74)	19% (35)	10% (31)
Research fellow or less	20% (35)	20% (51)	25% (28)

search centers we studied. When we consider both number of earlier socialization experiences and type of reaction to first socialization experience, we discover that both do interact with local rank in such a way that only the highest ranking members (Associate Attending or Attending) of the institutions can follow their own ethical bent. The relationship between socialization experiences and behavior does not appear at lower ranks. Similarly, those whose first reaction to the ethical issues of research was negative (in terms of the value of humane therapy) are less likely to engage in less fa-

Table 7.9.   Per Cent Engaged in Less Favorable Studies by Reaction to First
Awareness of Ethical Issues and Rank in Local Institution

Rank in Local Institution	*Reaction to First Awareness of Ethical Issues*		
	Negative	*Neutral*	*Positive*
Associate attending or Attending	17% (71)	17% (125)	32% (25)
Assistant attending	17% (41)	14% (102)	7% (14)
Research fellow or less	25% (36)	24% (110)	17% (12)

vorable studies than those whose first reaction was positive (in terms of the
value of research) only when we consider those of Associate Attending or
Attending rank.

Again, when we consider the per cent of researchers with differing
socialization experiences engaged in least favorable studies, the percentages
are, of course, reduced, but the differences observed in Tables 7.6–7.9 remain.
The data suggest that socialization and informal interaction structures, while
they may sometimes have direct and wholly independent effects on behavior,
also may have indirect or ·interdependent effects. They are both independent
and interdependent in bringing about effects. It may be that socialization results in dispositions to behave in certain ways toward research subjects, dispositions which will be activated to the extent that the individual researcher
is free to determine the conditions of his work.

8

SIX CASE STUDIES[1]

After an extended and detailed analysis in the last four chapters of the patterns, social sources, and consequences of conforming and deviant behavior in the use of human subjects, we will now provide some concrete examples of the abstract structures and processes we have delineated. We have seen how the dilemma of science and therapy, the competition structures of science in both the larger community and local institutions, socialization processes, and collaboration groups and informal interaction structures affect our aggregated data. How do such necessary and useful analytic structures reveal themselves in concrete individual cases? We hope to show how they do by presenting six individual case studies of research that clearly reveal the patterns we have discerned in our aggregate data. Each of the cases displays concretely one or more of the several analytic patterns we have already described in more abstract fashion.

These case studies do not constitute a representative sample of the research our respondents reported to us. In order to highlight the workings of our different explanatory variables, we discuss six studies that can be seen to be least favorable on our Risks–All Benefits Ratio, described in Chapter 3. The least favorable category includes all studies involving risk that is relatively high in proportion to anticipated therapeutic benefits for the subjects of the study itself, for any future patients, and/or for medical science in general.[2] We have seen, of course, that least favorable studies of this type are only an extremely small proportion of all biomedical research stud-

---

[1] It should be carefully noted that, in addition to these six least favorable cases there was a seventh one, which indeed was "the least favorable of all" and which does not seem to be explained by the patterns we have found to be helpful in the other six cases. Such a case shows the inevitable limits of the analysis as far as we have carried it. Such cases show too the need for further research and analysis.

[2] Although one of the six studies (Case 5) actually did not fall into this category in terms of the respondents' answers to questions about the risk-benefit ratio, it does seem to fall into this category when some side comments of the investigator are taken into account. That is, in regard to this study, the respondents volunteered information on the risk-benefit ratio in connection with other matters, rather than directly.

ies. But even this small proportion may have large consequences for a considerable number of subjects. And they are definitely the cases that present the most direct challenge to the fulfillment of the "humane therapy" value of biomedical researchers and to the effectiveness of social control procedures in this area. We have chosen the "problem" cases not to exaggerate their frequency but to focus on weaknesses in the existing structures of reward and control. Such a focus may strengthen the argument we present in the last chapter for needed changes in the present reward and control structures.

CASE 1 [3]

Our first example will really involve two studies by the same researcher which are very similar in method and goal. A young instructor mentioned in his interview that he was engaged in two studies with five other researchers. He indicated that, in both, he was the principal investigator. We eventually interviewed four of the five researchers he mentioned as collaborators, but none of them volunteered that they were involved in either of the studies in question. Four of the collaborators were very senior people and it may safely be assumed that they served more in a minimal consultative and sponsoring capacity than as active participants. This case suggests the need for such senior sponsors to look more carefully at the ethical aspects of studies they otherwise "approve." The fifth collaborator mentioned was more junior, and it is possible that he worked closely with the principal investigator, even though he also does not acknowledge participation in either study. We see here the fuzziness of affiliation we mentioned in the last chapter.

According to the principal investigator, the studies involved "some risk,"[4] in the form of catheterization, and no therapeutic benefit whatsoever to the subjects. He said that one of the studies would be a highly significant contribution to medical knowledge while the other would be a greater than average contribution. The first study would, he felt, result in some benefit to others in the future if successful, while the second study would result in no benefit to others in the future as far as he could see.

Seventy per cent of the subjects in the first study were ward patients in the hospital, while 80% of the subjects in the second study were ward patients. Note that a slightly higher percentage of ward patients was used

---

[3] An intensive effort has been made to conceal the actual identity of each of these researchers but nonetheless to preserve the verisimilitude of the actual research situation.

[4] It should be recalled here that "some risk," "moderate risk," and "large risk" fall into our highest category of risk for subject. See Chapter 3.

in the second study, which is less important scientifically and will result, even if successful, in no benefit to others in the future.

Though we did not ask our interviewees whether or not they were obtaining consent from their subjects, two comments by this researcher illustrate his probable attitude toward obtaining consent in his studies. Each respondent was asked:

> How often in the past year has the question of ethics come to your attention under each of the following circumstances?
> A. In connection with the practice of medicine? _____ times
> B. In connection with the use of human subjects in biomedical research? _____ times

In response to both parts of the question each interviewee was asked to give an example. This principal investigator gave an example from his own research:

> Whether or not a test or procedure with moderate risk and no therapeutic benefit for the subject should be done to him without his informed consent, especially in those cases where he will be billed for such procedures. We allow a number of these as long as there aren't too many, since there are no funds available for research we want to do.

Later in the interview schedule, also, there was a question which asked whether the respondent felt the present PHS policy on consent to be too restrictive. This investigator felt that it was "about right," but then commented:

> *De facto*, you inform the patient (even with respect to the details of risk, etc.), but you manipulate him through the way you present it. Especially in my field, you need subjects but they generally get little therapeutic benefit from the research. So, you have to appeal to their altruism, and if you're perfectly frank and honest you'll probably scare them away.

It is probably safe to assume that this research was not reviewed for its ethical aspects by this institution's peer review committee,[5] since it is hard to believe that the committee would sanction the policy of billing the patient for experimental procedures done on him without his consent.

This principal investigator chose the most permissive response to the bone metabolism hypothetical proposal, and the junior researcher he mentioned as a collaborator chose the next most permissive response.

While we have no definitive proof, it is likely that this junior collaborator, of all those mentioned, works closest with the principal investigator.

---

[5] In the next chapter we will present a detailed analysis of the structure and functioning of these local-institutional peer review committees.

While one of the two senior people mentioned also had a fairly permissive response, the remaining two gave the strictest response. One of them is one of the most senior men in his department, and he indicated in his interview that he presently does no research and is only peripherally involved with anyone else's research. His ability to know about the details of the research of junior people may be somewhat lessened because of this lack of contact. The same may be said of the other two senior people, both of whom are in a different department and may only have been minimally consulted by the young principal investigator.

The investigator in question here also exemplifies the extreme mass producer type. He has produced sixteen papers in the last five years, and he has received zero citations according to the data in the *Science Citation Index*. In addition, since he is at the lowest of the three levels of rank in his institution, he is also underrewarded when the sheer number of papers he has produced is considered.

CASE 2

This study involves the administration of a drug with potentially harmful side effects. According to the researcher there is "some risk" but only "minor" benefit for the subjects. In response to the question about the kinds of subjects involved in the study, moreover, the researcher indicated that even the minor benefit anticipated would apply to only 10% of the subjects. The remainder are patients who will receive no therapeutic benefits. So, for 90% of the subjects there is "some risk" and no therapeutic benefit. All subjects in the study are ward patients.

The researcher volunteered that, in his terms, he defined the study as *"ad hoc"* and that, therefore, he had not had it reviewed by his institution's peer review committee:

> I don't have too much experience with the committee, but it reviews what funded, formal research there is. My research, as I have said, is "ad hoc." This kind of research is not reviewed by the committee. I get around the committee. Quite a bit of such "ad hoc" research is carried on here; you don't need special funding for it.

The researcher views the study as a "modest, but important" contribution to medical knowledge and feels that it should result in "some" benefit to others in the future. There was one other named collaborator on the study, but he was affiliated with another local institution and, hence, was not interviewed.

In contrast to the previous case, this investigator was strict in his response to the bone metabolism hypothetical research proposal. He was unwilling to approve the study under any circumstances. How, then, do we find this investigator involved in a study of his own where the risks clearly outweigh the benefits to the subjects?

This researcher is 35 years old, involved in three research projects using human subjects, expressing concern about being anticipated, and has published twenty-five papers in the past five years while receiving zero citations to his work as recorded in the *Science Citation Index*. He is a clear example of our extreme mass producer type. According to our analysis he has been working very hard at trying to become an "established" researcher, but has had no success. He has been pressured, we infer, into taking short cuts. In addition, by our criteria, he is underrewarded when compared to his colleagues who have equal productivity of scientific papers. Ironically, he is taking risks with subjects on a study which not even he defines as really important scientifically. In his estimation the study will only be a "modest, but important" contribution if successful.

As the quotation about *ad hoc* research shows, this researcher was probably aware that his research violates the ethical standards prevalent in his institution. He was aware that all "funded, formal" research in his institution should be submitted to the peer review committee which would examine the ethical aspects of the research, but he chose to evade the requirement by saying that his research was only *ad hoc*. While apparently not violating the letter of the rules, he was certainly violating their spirit. A crucial structural condition for the existence of research of the kind analyzed so far must certainly be its invisibility. To the extent that a study is *ad hoc* so that it is not examined by the review committee, and is done on ward patients who are unlikely to protest or possibly even be informed that they are subjects, it can certainly be done more easily.

CASE 3

The next case is also a drug study. In this one a drug with fairly serious side effects for some people, but which has proved successful in the treatment of a certain disease, was being tried as a treatment for a totally different disease. Five investigators were collaborating in this study and we interviewed four of them. Three of the four that we interviewed acknowledged their participation in the study, while the fourth indicated that he was collaborating on two other studies with this group but not on this one. The person who was not interviewed was the overall director of the larger research program, but the principal investigator on this particular part of the program was one of those we did interview.

According to the principal investigator, the study involves a "moderate" amount of risk and "some" benefit to the subjects if successful. The other two researchers who acknowledged participation in the study, and hence gave us data about it, said that the study involved "very little" risk. One said that there would be "little or no" benefit if the study was successful, while the other said "minor" benefit.

The principal investigator and one other collaborator gave the most permissive response to the bone metabolism hypothetical research proposal. They would approve the study with only a 10% chance of success. Another said he would approve it if the chance of success were 50%. The fourth collaborator that we interviewed gave the strictest response. He would not approve the study as stated regardless of the chance for success.

The fourth collaborator is an interesting case. He indicated in his interview that he was in conflict with his collaborators about the value of the drug being tested and had considered leaving the project. He felt that the drug was of no value, but he indicated that the study would be a "highly significant contribution" even if the drug was proven worthless, since the drug would then not be used as a treatment for the disease being studied. He said that he knew the study would proceed without him if he left, and so he felt he could do more good by staying on. The other two researchers who gave data on the study, those who were permissive in the response to the hypothetical proposal, indicated that in their view the study would be a "modest, but important" contribution. Again, a risky study with low benefit for subjects is defined by the investigators as of low scientific value. Finally, in this study 100% of the subjects were ward patients.

Interestingly, all three of the researchers interviewed who acknowledged participation in this drug study indicated in response to another question that there had been many discussions with the others over ethical dilemmas arising out of the research. Two of them said that they had had such discussions with the others 20 to 25 times in the past year. For all three the issue was the same: should a subject who experiences bad side effects from the drug be withdrawn from the study? Though we do not know who took what side in the issue, we do know that the researcher with the strictest standards mentioned being in conflict with the others over the value of the drug. This is an example of the kind of intercolleague influence that can take place after the study commences. To the extent that the strict researcher has been able to exert any influence on the others, the subjects will have benefited.

The principal investigator in this study, whom we have already described as being permissive in his response to our hypothetical research proposal, is also underrewarded when compared to his colleagues who have equal productivity and equal citations. He is also a graduate of an elite medical school. That he may perhaps feel pressure to move too quickly in his research may be inferred from the following statement where he indicates his past and present impatience with the peer review process in his institution:

> One of my proposals was delayed (by the peer review committee). I feel unnecessarily, because of a clinical psychologist's own personal bad experience with or fear of spinal taps, plus his lack of knowledge because he was not a physician. Also, there have been cases of "hamstringing" proposals because of professional jealousies.

In addition, two of the three investigators who acknowledge participation in the study are moderately concerned about being anticipated in this research. The third, the strict collaborator, is only slightly concerned about the possibility of being anticipated. Being aware of the existence of competitors must certainly have the effect of putting pressure on the researchers not to eliminate from the study subjects who experience side effects.

CASE 4

As with all but one of the previous cases, the study to be presented now is a drug study. Two researchers are involved, and both were interviewed. Both acknowledge doing the study and each chooses the other. The principal investigator is slightly more senior than the other investigator, and the junior investigator says that it is his first study.

The junior investigator says that the study involves "some" risk and "minor" benefit to the subjects, while the principal investigator says "very little" risk and "little or no" benefit. Upon inspection of both investigators' responses to an earlier question about the characteristics of the subjects, however, it is revealed that some 70–80% of the subjects are exposed to possibly as much as "some" risk and it is expected that they will receive no therapeutic benefit since they are normal controls. The principal investigator says that, if successful, the study will be a "highly significant" contribution to medical knowledge and will result in "some" therapeutic benefit to others in the future. The junior investigator disagrees, saying that it will be a "greater than average" contribution but will probably result in only "minor" therapeutic benefit to patients in the future.

In addition, one of the investigators said that 99% of the subjects are ward patients. The other said that 80% are from the ward. In any event, the large majority of the subjects are ward patients.

The principal investigator in the study, as in most of the previous cases, gave the most permissive response to the bone metabolism hypothetical research proposal that we presented interviewees for review. The junior collaborator said that he could justify the bone metabolism hypothetical study only if the chances of success were at least 90%

In addition to being permissive in his ethical standards, the principal investigator is also underrewarded when it comes to his research quality and quantity. This researcher has received a total of 48 citations to his work, four times the mean number for those researchers in the highest ranks of the institution, and he has published 20 papers in the past five years but he is still an assistant professor. He is also from an elite medical school. Though he is only 35 years old,[6] and hence on grounds of seniority may not be as eligible for promotion as some, he ranks in the top 5% of our sample of researchers on number of citations. In a system that rewards quality of research very highly, he would have to be at the top. We have here, then, a willing personality that is, in addition, being subjected to two kinds of pressures: the need to perform well enough to be promoted locally and the need to perform fast enough so that his competitors do not publish first.

The junior investigator, though strict in his response to our hypothetical question and not an extreme mass producer, stresses that he has learned the need to publish often and quickly in order to obtain advancement. He has also clearly been socialized by his colleagues more strongly to accept the values of science than the values of humane therapy:

> When you find out the way you're going to make a name and a position for yourself is by publishing, you shift your prejudice from one side to another.

CASE 5

Another study, according to the investigator, involved "some" risk for the subjects and would involve "some" benefit for 90% of the subjects if successful and "no" benefit for 10% who served as controls. The 90% were "patients for whom the investigation may have eventual therapeutic benefits, but who are primarily subjects of scientific research." The study was intended to determine the effect of a drug on a major body organ, and a catheter would be inserted into the organ as part of the design. About half of the subjects were ward patients. This is the study, referred to in footnote 2, which was not included as least favorable in our Risks–All Benefits Ratio but which, on the basis of additional information given us by the investigator, really belongs here.

Three investigators were involved in the study, and we interviewed two

---

[6] Thirty-five is not young for an assistant professor in an arts and science faculty, but many researchers have four years of medical school, one year of internship, three years of residency, and one to three years of postdoctoral research training at the rank of research fellow. This means that a researcher could be as old as 31 or 32 before being eligible for an assistant professorship.

of them including the principal investigator. The principal investigator, though chosen as a collaborator, did not acknowledge his participation in the study when interviewed. Our data on the study's characteristics, therefore, come only from the investigator who reported participation in the study. This lack of acknowledgement often occurred in our study when the person chosen as principal investigator had merely obtained funds or was the overall but remote supervisor. He viewed his role as only tangential to particular projects, while his subordinates viewed him as the principal investigator. Again we suggest, the role of principal investigator may require better control than it now receives.

The principal investigator chose the most permissive choice on the bone metabolism hypothetical proposal, and the other investigator we interviewed chose the next most permissive alternative. The second investigator would approve the hypothetical study if there were only a 30% chance of success, while the principal investigator would approve it if there were a 10% chance of success. The junior investigator, though not literally an extreme mass producer, certainly comes close to representing that type. In the past five years he had produced fourteen papers and one book, but he had received only two citations to his life's work as recorded in the *Science Citation Index*. The principal investigator was also slightly concerned about the possibility of being anticipated, and we have commented elsewhere on the way in which the awareness of competition might foster impatience in a researcher. This case, then, is another example of a now familiar theme.

CASE 6

This sixth example also shows concretely the applicability of our analysis. Three investigators, all of whom we interviewed, were involved in a study which, according to the principal investigator, involved "some" risk and "minor" benefit for subjects. Only the principal investigator acknowledged participation in this study, and though he chose the other two as collaborators he indicated that they were really more consultants than collaborators. This could explain why they did not list themselves as collaborators.

The experimental procedure involved a biopsy in children. Though the principal investigator indicated that the study would involve "minor" benefit, 50% of the subjects were children with conditions unrelated to the investigation and were to serve as controls. The other 50% were "patients for whom the investigation may have *eventual* therapeutic benefits, but who are primarily subjects of scientific research." So, in fact, at least 50% of the subjects would be subject to "some" risk but would receive no benefit whatsoever. The investigator also defined the study as likely to be only a "modest, but important" contribution if successful, but he anticipated "some" benefit for others in the future if the study worked out as he planned. Ninety-five per cent of the subjects were ward patients.

This investigator's response to the bone metabolism hypothetical proposal was fairly strict. He said that the study should be approved only if it had a 90% chance of success. However, on the pulmonary function hypothetical proposal, the principal investigator stated that consent "should not be obtained" from subjects undergoing pulmonary function tests under anesthesia for hernia repair. Even though anesthesia would be extended for an additional half-hour just to complete the study, this investigator felt that consent should not be obtained for participation in the study. Thus, though this investigator was not permissive as measured by the bone metabolism hypothetical proposal, he did have permissive standards with respect to the consent issue as measured by his response to the pulmonary function hypothetical proposal. He was also nearly an extreme mass producer with eleven papers and only two citations, and he was also slightly concerned about being anticipated.

When we asked this investigator for comments about his experiences with the institutional review committee, he said: "No personal experience. I try to avoid having my research reviewed."

This researcher was also one of those who was classified in our analysis of socialization as having a strong belief in the "value of research." He states that his research experiences have led him to believe that the knowledge which results from research justifies taking risks with patients:

> [As I gained more experience in research] I became more aggressive, less conservative. I became convinced that research helps knowledge, and I therefore weighted ethical issues less. I have never encountered a bad result in my own research of a kind that would make me more conservative. . . .
>
> The only subject in the end is the human himself. My conviction that research will increase knowledge allowed me to take risks with patients.

It is ironic, of course, that he himself defines this particular study as likely to involve only "modest, but important" results, a low estimate of scientific significance according to our scale.

We now present an additional concrete illustration of some of the abstract findings of our previous chapters. This example is a very short "professional biography" derived from our interview with a young biomedical researcher. This biography provides us with an opportunity to see the processes and development over time of the ethical standards and practices of clinical investigators. Our six cases were more static, without the processual quality that is revealed here:

> As new medical students, he and his peers [probably identifying with the

patient-subjects] were prejudiced against the clinical investigator in cases of difficult ethical issues. As an intern with patients wanted by investigators, he was confronted with pondering the ethical issues, because now these were patients for whose welfare he was responsible. When he began to do his own research as a resident, he still saw things more as a physician than a researcher and was shocked at the tactics researchers used to get consent from subjects. When he became a research fellow, he was told by his senior-researcher mentor to get informed consent from subjects, and he rather scrupulously tried to do so. But he soon learned of the actual practice in this respect when he saw his senior researcher-mentor "sell" a patient on becoming a subject by "stretching the truth" about the potential benefits the patient might hope for. Also, he realized that his rewards as a researcher lay in publishing, and that his more honest, detailed, informing of patients rather frequently resulted in their refusal to be subjects so that it would take him longer to do studies (if he could get enough subjects to do them at all) and, therefore, to gain a name and advancement. His attitudes changed from being prejudiced against the researcher to being prejudiced in his favor, as his role, self-image, and rewards changed. In retrospect, he now sees his earlier attitudes as somewhat naive. Now he feels he understands better the importance of good medical research, even, at times, when there is no potential benefit for the subjects themselves. Also, he feels he is more balanced in his decisions regarding scientific advance as weighed against the rights and welfare of subjects than he was when he judged researchers and their research as a medical student. He will not "sell" patients on becoming subjects by lying or stretching the truth. But, if important research is to get done and he is to publish, "salesmanship" is necessary. He feels it is more ethical salesmanship to gain rapport with the patient, to get the patient's confidence, and to tell the patient about discomforts and very generally about risks and benefits, but ultimately to ask the patient to trust him.

So much, then, for the way in which our six concrete cases and one "biography" vividly illustrate the structures, processes, social determinants, and ethical consequences that we have reported more abstractly in earlier chapters. We now turn to a final phase of this abstract analysis, the last of our types of social control: peer group review.

9

SOCIAL CONTROL: THE STRUCTURES, PROCESSES, AND EFFICACY OF PEER GROUP REVIEW

We return now to our more systematic and abstract analysis. In this chapter we deal with the last of our three types of social control, peer group review, which is a set of formally defined structures and processes that various governmental (e.g., the P.H.S. and the F.D.A.) and individual biomedical research organizations have stipulated as necessary for producing normatively desirable social performance with regard to the use of human subjects by their grantees or members. This is the type of relevant social control where probably the largest changes have occurred in recent years and with probably the most consequential effects. First, we shall present a brief history of the evolution of peer group review structures and processes, together with a description of their present operation based on data from our National Survey. Then, in the latter part of the chapter, we shall proceed to an evaluation of the efficacy of the new arrangements.

We may recall from Chapter 2 that the data analyzed in this chapter were collected in our National Survey, a mail questionnaire study of a nationally representative sample of biomedical research institutions using human subjects. The questionnaires were filled out most commonly by the institution's director of research, a senior official who was also most commonly himself a research physician. In most cases the respondent seems to have had considerable assistance from his colleagues and staff. The questions asked in our National Survey focused predominantly on peer group review.

HISTORY AND EVOLUTION OF PEER GROUP REVIEW

We start with a brief history of the development of formal peer group review of biomedical research on human subjects and a short account of its present legal and administrative status. Above all, the recency of this development must be kept in mind. Peer review is an important social invention, but an invention that has not yet had time to take even near final shape and to give more than perhaps only satisfactory performance. As is the case also with written codes of ethics for such matters, peer review committees and procedures are pretty much a product of the late 1950's and the 1960's. As Professor William J. Curran, a pioneer in the field, has said, "the need to identify and develop acceptable standards of care (for human subjects) . . . began to receive limited but respectable support in the clinical research community in the late 1950's and early 1960's."[1] When Dr. Louis Welt, a practicing physician, sent a questionnaire to every university department of medicine in the country in 1960 asking them whether they had "a procedural document dealing with problems of human experimentation" and whether they favored "a committee of disinterested faculty . . . [to] review the experimental design to insure maximum protection for the subject," he received replies from 66 of the approximately 80 existing departments.[2] "Of these," he reported, "only eight have a procedural document and only twenty-four have or favor a committee to review problems in human experimentation."[3] Just a little later, the newly established Law-Medicine Research Institute at Boston University, with a grant approved and funded by the National Institutes of Health, did a similar study.[4] This Institute survey of 86 departments of medicine produced 52 responses which gave much the same results as the Welt survey. Only 9 departments had procedural documents, with 5 more indicating that they were in process of developing one or favored doing so. Twenty-two of the departments reported that they had peer review committees but that these were only "advisory." In sum, as Curran has put it, "it is evident that in the medical research community prior to 1962 there was a general skepticism toward the development of ethical guidelines, codes, or sets of procedures concerning the conduct of research."[5] Furthermore, "it was the posture of both the FDA and the NIH to allow and to encourage clinical investigators . . . to be guided by their own professional judgment and controlled by their own ethical standards as well as those of their institutions."[6]

In the early 1960's, a series of public events and official actions transformed the whole environment for controls on the use of human subjects. From 1959 to 1962, Senator Kefauver's hearings brought the problem of the possible abuse of human subjects, as well as many other drug abuses, before public attention. These hearings, supported by the public horror at the news

---

[1] William J. Curran, "Governmental Regulation of the Use of Human Subjects in Medical Research: The Approach of Two Federal Agencies," *Daedalus*, 98, no. 2 (Spring, 1969): 545.

[2] Louis G. Welt, "Reflections on the Problems of Human Experimentation," *Connecticut Medicine*, 25 (1961): 75–78.

[3] *Ibid.*

[4] Curran, *op. cit.*, pp. 545–594.

[5] *Ibid.*, p. 548.

[6] *Ibid.*

of the thalidomide tragedy in Germany, resulted in the Drug Amendment Acts of 1962, one of the provisions of which was the first grant of statutory authority for control in these matters. The Food and Drug Administration was now required to see that all human subjects were asked to sign a patient consent form. Another cause célèbre, the Southam and Mandel case in New York State in which live cancer cells were injected into geriatric patients without their informed consent, contributed to the growing climate of increased attention and concern (see Chapter 1, footnote 9). After much consultation with the clinical research community, in 1966 Commissioner Goddard of the F.D.A. issued a detailed *Statement of Policy Concerning Consent.*

Another and very important event in the development of procedural controls came in the same year when the Public Health Service issued its first statement on "Protection of the Individual as a Research Subject," which has been under continuous revision since its initial formulation.[7] Most recently, for example, the P.H.S. has required that all proposals for funds from P.H.S. for research using human subjects be screened by peer review "prior to submission to the Public Health Service," not after a grant has been given, as was the case up to then.[8] Because the P.H.S. funds a considerable proportion of the biomedical research conducted in the United States, because this regulation is therefore applicable to just about all American biomedical research institutions, and because its guidelines for control by a peer review committee are broad and inclusive, it is this regulation that has been so consequential for the peer group review process. The peer review committee is instructed to look to three problems in every piece of research using human subjects which is supported by P.H.S. funds: (1) the rights and welfare of the subject; (2) the appropriateness of the methods of getting consent; and (3) the risks and potential benefits of the investigation.[9]

---

[7] For an intensive history of the evolution and development of the P.H.S. policy since 1953, see Mark S. Frankel, *The Public Health Service Guidelines Governing Research Involving Human Subjects: An Analysis of the Policy-Making Process* (Washington, D.C.: Program of Policy Studies in Science and Technology, The George Washington University), February, 1972.

[8] According to our National Survey, which began before this new requirement was officially circulated among institutions by P.H.S., the timing of peer review of clinical research proposals for funds from P.H.S. was, in actual practice in institutions, as follows: 69% of our respondents claimed that in their institutions such proposals were reviewed only before application to P.H.S.; on the other hand, just 4% admitted to review only after funding had been approved by P.H.S.; the remaining 27% reported a review prior to funding but after application to P.H.S., or some combination of this, review before application, and review after funding.

[9] Eugene A. Confrey, "Public Health Service-Supported Research Involving Human Subjects" (unpublished paper given at the Conference on the Ethical Aspects of Experimentation on Human Subjects, sponsored by *Daedalus* and the National Institutes of Health, Boston, Nov., 1967).

In 1971, the F.D.A. added the requirement of peer review for all clinical research presented to it by drug companies. And also in 1971, the Department of Health, Education and Welfare, parent organization of N.I.H. and P.H.S., declared that, in principle, all *non*medical research supported by its funds was also to be subject to peer review. The principle of peer review has come a long way in a short time.

Some results of our National Survey of biomedical research institutions using human subjects (institutions drawn from the May 1969, P.H.S. list of assurances given) round out and support the picture drawn thus far of the development of peer review.[10] Because so many of such institutions took its grants, the P.H.S. regulation had a large and immediate effect. Fifty-four per cent of the institutions reported that they had filed assurances of compliance in 1966, another 28% had done so in 1967, and the other 18% had taken action in 1968 or 1969. We also asked our respondents whether there was "a review procedure which scrutinized the ethical aspects of proposed clinical research before the National Institutes of Health required that one be put into effect." Some 70% reported that they had had a review procedure. Since this is somewhat larger than the 36% reported in the Welt study and the 42% reported in the Law-Medicine Research Institute study having or favoring peer review, it would seem that there had been a gradual increase in the nonrequired review procedures and committees from 1960 to 1966.[11] However, in 38% of those institutions which reported to us that they already had review procedures when the P.H.S. regulation was put into effect in 1966, the previously existing procedures were found, to some greater or lesser degree, not to measure up to the new P.H.S. standards. That is, this 38% also reported to us that P.H.S. had required them to make major (12%) or minor (26%) changes in their review procedures to make them acceptable under its 1966 regulation. Moreover, another 24% of these institutions with previous review procedures reported that, although no revisions had been required by P.H.S., they had taken the opportunity to make some changes in the procedures on their own. The new regulation thus both brought new committees into being and caused the procedures of previously established committees to be improved.

Now that peer review committees are probably universally established

---

[10] The findings which follow are based on the returns of the 293 institutions which responded in our National Survey. For a full discussion of the methodological aspects of the National Survey, see Chapter 2.

[11] Even if, in order to replicate more closely the Welt and the Law-Medicine Research Institute studies which surveyed university departments of medicine, we consider only the percentage of medical schools which reported to us that they had had previous review procedures—51% ($N = 57$)—there still seems to have been gradual progress from 1960 to 1966.

in biomedical research institutions, how wide is the scope of their control over the research using human subjects done in their home institutions? How many researchers can validly claim, "In our institution *all* research using human subjects is reviewed"? Looking for data on the scope of control that peer review committees now exercise, in our National Survey study we asked our respondents to tell us whether "all clinical research" was reviewed, or "only clinical research which involves a formal proposal for funds, either for funds from your institution's research budget or for funds from an external institution or agency" or, finally, "only formal proposals to do clinical research which involve requests for money from the Public Health Service." Eighty-five per cent of the institutions responded that "all clinical research" was now reviewed. Another 10% said that only clinical research which involves a formal proposal for funds from whatever source was reviewed. And 5% said that only formal proposals to the P.H.S. are reviewed. Our data in-indicate that 35%(43) of the institutions where less than all clinical research is reviewed are medical schools, that is, generally the type of institutional setting most productive of biomedical investigations using human subjects. It is clear then that a perhaps significant volume of human research is still not subject to review by peer review committees.

Evidence from our interviewing of biomedical researchers at University Hospital and Research Center and at Community and Teaching Hospital indicates that even in institutions where there is a peer review committee presumably reviewing all clinical research, there is another perhaps important minority of research activities which is not submitted to peer review. At University Hospital and Research Center 8% (325) and at Community and Teaching Hospital 9% (55) of the researchers we interviewed *volunteered* the information that one or more of their investigations using human subjects had not been reviewed by the peer review committee. A few more informed us that they knew of what they called "ad hoc" or "nonsystematic" human research by others which was not reviewed by the committee.

Knowledge of such violations or evasions immediately raises the question whether there is need to institute some policing procedure.[12] Moreover, those who volunteered this information about unreviewed research by themselves or others indicated two structured sources for such bypassing of the review committee, and knowledge of these sources suggests other remedies. First, what is considered "delay" in the reviewing process may generate evasion techniques. At University Hospital and Research Center, it takes about a month from the time a protocol is submitted to the time it is

---

[12] Kenneth L. Melmon, Michael Grossman, and R. Curtis Morris, Jr., "Emerging Assets and Liabilities of a Committee on Human Welfare and Experimentation," *The New England Journal of Medicine*, 282 (1970): 427–431.

considered by the review committee. Researchers racing to establish priority of discovery or those who feel that some case or situation presents them with "now or never" opportunities to do research may both feel that this is an unacceptably long time to wait.[13] Instead of waiting, they go ahead without submitting a protocol for review at all or, alternatively, submit a protocol but go ahead before it is approved. Recognizing this structure of *experienced* "delay" as one source of evasion of review, the review committees at the University of California Medical School in San Francisco are required to complete their reports within 10 days. At this institution, and perhaps elsewhere, there is also provision for immediate administrative review in exceptional cases.[14] Procedures for especially speedy review where the researchers are afraid of undue delay would probably be necessary only in a minority of cases and would cut down the evasion that is caused by these exigencies in biomedical research.

A second structural source of evasion of, or indifference to, peer review procedures arises from the genuine and not infrequent ambiguity regarding what is "clinical research" and what is a small, everyday variation on standard medical or surgical procedures. Evidence on this ambiguity is available in the responses to a question we asked in our National Survey. We asked our respondents whether the following definition of clinical research was "personally acceptable to you without addition or deletion":

> *Clinical Research or Investigation:* Anything done to a person which is as yet not established, by clinical experience or scientific research, as being for his direct therapeutic benefit or as contributing to the diagnosis of his disease. (What is done may eventually, of course, be for the person's own direct or indirect therapeutic benefit and/or for the eventual therapeutic benefit of the population at large.) Investigations which involve the analysis of human substances collected as a by-product of established diagnostic or other procedures should be included here as clinical research.

While 76% of our respondents agreed with this definition, the rest did not. Those who disagreed with our definition suggested alternative definitions. Some were more inclusive than ours, and some were more exclusive. Until definitional ambiguities are reduced, it is inevitable that a certain amount of clinical research may not be defined as such and may be carried out without peer review.

Let us turn now to a description of the present structure and processes of the peer review committee. A better understanding of these matters will help us better understand how effectively the committee makes decisions and carries out its functions.

As might be expected from the recency of its development, and as the

---

[13] On the importance of priority in research, see Merton, "Priorities...."
[14] See Melmon, et al., *op. cit.*, p. 428.

data from our National Survey indeed confirm, the peer review group in its typical structure is still not highly differentiated or specialized.[15] One of the questions we asked our respondents was, "Is the institutional review committee itself specialized in any way into subcommittees, departmental committees, or an executive committee; or, are there other review committees dealing with the ethical aspects of clinical research in your institution?" Sixty-eight per cent of the respondents said their peer review committees were not specialized in any way. Fifteen per cent indicated that there were other review committees in their institutions, either at some higher or lower level of the structure or at some affiliated institution. Only 10% report specialization into subcommittees, and only 4% report specialized departmental committees. Only 8% of the institutions have executive committees for their peer review groups. Only 5% of the institutions claim that they have any members at all who spend "full time" in the activities of the peer review committee.

As might be further expected from such relatively undifferentiated groups, the number of members is typically small. Twenty-seven per cent of the institutions reported 1 to 5 members; another 48% reported 6 to 10; and 25% report more than 10, with only one institution reporting as many as 40 members on its review committee. (One institution reported that currently there were no committee members.)

It may be useful here to note that authorities at the University of California San Francisco Medical Center believe that a single stable committee, small enough to be of manageable size, cannot possess talents diverse enough to allow meaningful review, considering the wide range of subject matter involved in the large number of research applications submitted by Medical Center researchers. For this reason, the committee established itself as parent group to three-man *ad hoc* review committees whom it specifically selected for each research protocol submitted. Among the conclusions of a study of the first two years of operation of the committee under this system is the following:

> We believe that slow rotation of the membership of the [parent committee], slow progress of a member to chairmanship, and overlapping terms of service will provide consistency in policy. We strongly endorse the ad hoc committee concept both for its flexibility in providing the best reviewers for each situation and for continuously and painlessly expanding the number of faculty informed on and concerned with policy on investigation in human beings.[16]

A further indication of the lack of differentiation in peer review group

---

[15] Not surprisingly also, our data suggest that differentiation and specialization—or lack of it—of the committee is partly a function of the number and variety of clinical research proposals to be reviewed in an institution.

[16] Melmon, et al., *op. cit.*, pp. 428, 431.

structure is the admixture of other functions besides that of ethical review. In 22% of the responding institutions, for example, the peer review committee also allocates the institution's research funds to its clinical investigators. In two-thirds of our sample, the peer review committee also evaluates the scientific merit of proposed clinical research. Since scientific merit (e.g., representativeness and size of sample) are often related to ethical issues (e.g., too small a sample merely puts subjects at risk unnecessarily, too large a sample may put too many subjects at risk), it is often not desirable to separate the reviewing of ethical and scientific issues. But insofar as a committee is not relating scientific merit to ethical concerns, its lack of differentiation may reduce its competence with either one of these two issues. One informant even told us that his peer review committee reviewed the cost-effectiveness of all proposed researches. While again this may sometimes be related to ethical matters, it is often quite another and related issue which should be left to other committees.

As to rank of peer review committee members in the formal hierarchy of their institutions, here again the typical structure seems to be less differentiated than it might be. Four-fifths of the institutions report that most of the members of their peer review committees come from the highest level of the formal institutional hierarchy, including the clinical, administrative, and academic. In the other institutions, the majority of the peer review members are from the intermediate level. Nowhere is a majority from the lower levels. A different mixture of members from different levels might give the peer review committees a more differentiated set of viewpoints on the ethical issues they are required to screen.

Finally, the relative lack of differentiation of the structure of review committees is manifest in the categories of types of activities, specialties, and occupational roles that their members are selected from. Here we discuss only actual members of peer review committees. Although at least some committees also use consultants, we do not have systematic data on this practice.

First, we consider committee members who belong to the local institution. There is a heavy emphasis on members with experience in clinical research, as there of course needs to be, though perhaps somewhat too much so at the expense of other types of members who have other knowledge and viewpoints to bring to the decisions of the committee. Thirteen per cent of the responding institutions report that they have *only* personnel of their own who engage in clinical research on their peer review committees. Overall, 93% of the institutions report members from among those on their staffs who actually engage in clinical investigations. Thirty per cent report M.D. members who do not do clinical research. Forty-three per cent report that they have pathologists as members. Sixty per cent report administrators as members, probably in recognition of the administrative responsibility of the institution for complying with P.H.S. regulations. Eighteen per cent say that nurses are members. And then there is a scattering of those employed by the institution in other types of roles: 9% have lawyers employed by the institution as members; 9%, members of the board of trustees; 9%, basic scientists; 9%, so-called "behavioral scientists" (a term that includes social scientists, psychologists, and social workers); and 2%, pharmacologists or pharmacists.

As for "outsiders" of various kinds, that is, those who are either clinical research specialists or physicians in other institutions or those who have nonmedical roles in the larger community and who are not in the employ of the institution, the typical peer review committee has small place for them as members. Only 10% of the responding institutions said they had members on their peer review committees from other institutions who do clinical research in the general areas in which members of the institution do research and 10% use M.D.'s from other institutions who do no clinical research in the institution's areas of specialization. Only 4% use outside lawyers; only 5% use outside "behavioral scientists"; and only 4% use clergymen. Only one institution has a patient sitting on its peer review committee. Finally, only 22% altogether of the institutions have *any kind* of outsider (in this sense of nonmember of the institution) as a committee member. Some institutions do use outside consultants but, again, we do not have data on this practice. Thus, very few peer review committees use outsiders as regular members either to bring them kinds of expertise they might want or, even more importantly, to provide the universalistic standards that may often be hard for members of a particular institution to apply to one another just because they are caught up inevitably in a web of personal and particularistic relationships with many of their colleagues.

While speaking of mechanisms to help insure universalistic application of standards in review of protocols, we should mention a finding by Melmon and his colleagues in their study of the peer review committee for the University of California San Francisco Medical Center.

> Most of the reviewers interviewed believed that protocols should be submitted anonymously; some admitted that they were swayed by the academic status of the investigator. A distinct minority admitted that incomplete protocols were more likely to be passed if submitted by a full professor with a "good reputation" than if submitted by a younger, "less established" faculty member.[17]

As an additional aid to universalism, these authors also recommend use of randomization in the selection of *ad hoc* subcommittees of experts which evaluate each protocol under the direction of the parent committee.[18]

---

[17] Melmon, et al., *op. cit.*, p. 430.
[18] *Ibid.*, p. 431.

Given this relatively undifferentiated structure of the typical peer review committee, what does our National Survey tell us about some of the typical processes and amounts of review that such a committee engages in? We were interested, first, in the intensiveness of the review process, so we asked if there were any kinds of pre-review before the whole committee met and we also asked if indeed the whole committee did meet. Seventy-five per cent of the respondents reported some kind of pre-review, that is, by all the individual members, or by a few of them, or by at least one. This procedure is obviously a more intensive kind of review than that engaged in by the 14% of the committees that reported no pre-review at all before the committee met as a whole. Further, 11% of our respondents indicate other procedures, frequently ones in which the committee does not meet as a body. Instead, for example, one or more individual members perform the review and a decision is reached after communication among the chairman and the members by phone or mail only. In such cases, the degree of intensiveness of consideration which might come from face-to-face interaction among the members of the peer review committee is obviously lacking.

In that large majority (92%) of the responding institutions where the committee at least sometimes met as a body, either with or without pre-review, a varying number of meetings was required to handle the work load. Fifty-five per cent of these committees that met as a body came together 1 to 10 times a year; 38% met 11 times or more (the greatest frequency being, in one case, 52 times); and 7% were indefinite, indicating only that they came together "as required." Of the committees meeting as a body, 35% reported an average of fewer than two proposals considered per meeting; 41% indicated 2 to 3.9 proposals; and 24% reported 4 or more proposals (the maximum number being, in one institution, 40). Obviously, the workload of a peer review committee can vary considerably.

Since the degree of consensus among those who interact with one another is always an important sociological variable, we were, of course, especially interested in discovering what degree of consensus the members of a peer review committee required of themselves in coming to a decision about the ethical propriety of a research protocol. Therefore we asked what proportion of the membership so voting is required for approval or disapproval of a protocol. Forty-two per cent of the responding institutions said their procedures required unanimity; 26%, a simple majority; 5%, a two-thirds majority; and 27% had no specific proportion stipulated in their procedure. These data show some considerable tendency toward that large degree of consensus, even toward unanimity, that we expect from groups that define themselves as "collegial," that is, as a company of near-equals sharing a single set of values, rather than as "political," that is, a group of unequals with divergent values and interests. In the former group, there would be a greater tendency to unanimity; in the latter, a simple majority would tend to be adequate for deciding among somewhat different interests and values.

This expected tendency to unanimity is even more clearly revealed in the responses to another question. We approached the unanimity tendency more directly when we asked:

> Do you agree or disagree with the following: "In practice, when our institutional review committee approves a clinical research proposal, it is almost always by a unanimous decision. If even one member has serious questions about the ethical aspects of such a proposal, we would probably either table the discussion, require revisions to satisfy the dissenting members, or even reject the proposal."

In only 4% of the cases does the respondent report that he disagrees with this statement. Ninety-one per cent agree with it (4% say they don't know), thus indicating the great tendency toward unanimity that one would expect in collegial groups making decisions about matters that are clearly of vital importance to their shared fundamental values. Even though the formal rules stated in their written procedures most often do not require unanimity, the informal sociological pressures toward unanimity are great enough to make it the nearly universal norm.

The Public Health Service Regulation, "Protection of the Individual as a Research Subject," requires not only an initial review of all research protocols but also continuing review.[19] The Regulation states that "the committee shall carry out interim review of all research in such a manner and at appropriate intervals in the light of apparent risks, existing administrative and supervisory organization, and other factors as to assure itself that its advice is being followed." How well did the typical review committee follow this mandate for continuing review of its approval-decisions? (It should be noted that this mandate was not officially circulated by the P.H.S. until after the majority of our questionnaires came in. However, this mandate had been proposed earlier and our respondents' institutions should have been aware of it.) Not too well, seems to be the answer given by our respondents. Twenty-three per cent of the responding institutions reported no continuing review at all. Only 36% claimed continuing formal review by the committee. Another 3% indicated interim review by the committee if it was notified of variance from the protocol originally approved. Thirty-two per cent reported wholly or partly informal continuing review. Six per cent reported that interim review was given not by the peer review committee but by some institutional officials, such as department heads. The lack of wholly satisfactory continuing review is further evident in the fact that some of the institutions claiming continuing review, formal or informal, indicated in

---

[19] See P.H.S. pamphlet, May 1, 1969.

their responses to our request to be specific about what this continuing review consisted in that it was fairly perfunctory or operated only in some cases, not in all. For example, a few respondents indicated that continuing review consisted in "informal discussion at lunch," or "through personal contact with researchers," or "as concern arises on the part of investigator, administrator, or senior faculty member." It is evident that procedures and practices for continuing review will have to be strengthened in many biomedical research institutions using human subjects. Of course, it should be carefully noted that even efficacious review of clinical research as it is proposed, without some kind of effective review of that research *as it is being carried out in practice,* does not guarantee adequate protection of human subjects.

One last aspect of the review committee decision process remains to be examined. In well-differentiated systems for making adjudicatory decisions, there is some mechanism for those whose cases are being adjudicated to make an appeal from what they consider erroneous decisions. In this respect, again, we find that the review committee system has not moved all the way toward adequate functional differentiation. In response to our question on this matter, only 46% of the responding institutions reported that they have any formal procedure by which a negative decision can be appealed from the review committee to some other body. This situation in which the majority of biomedical research institutions have not yet set up an appeal procedure as part of their peer review apparatus may be having negative consequences both for acceptance of peer review and for the progress of medical science. We have heard researchers object to peer review as they know or understand it because they believe that research proposals having real potential for medical scientific advances, or even "pioneering breakthroughs," frequently either are not or will not be approved by those who sit on institutional review committees. The reasons for these rejections they are especially concerned about do not involve the ethical defectiveness of the proposals. Rather they include local institutional politics and conflicts as well as resistance to innovations just because they depart from accustomed ways of scientific thinking and proceeding.[20] Indeed, to forestall rejections of this kind the biomedical community may have to go beyond the establishment of local appeal procedures by institutions. Perhaps what is necessary is the establishment of a hierarchy of "courts of appeal" throughout the nation, culminating, as a final resort, in a "supreme court" composed of eminent peers including both "insiders" and "outsiders" with respect to any field. Such a

---

[20] See Bernard Barber, "Resistance by Scientists to Scientific Discovery," *Science,* 134 (1961): 596–602, and T. S. Kuhn, *The Structure of Scientific Revolutions* (Chicago: University of Chicago Press, 1962).

system might be the best safeguard available against the object of these concerns—unjustified hindrance of medical progress by the peer review process.

Finally in regard to group structure and process, we asked the respondent for each institution in our survey:

> In addition to the review committee, are there any other institutional controls, formal or informal, over the ethical aspects of clinical research in your institution? (For example: the department chairman may have to review proposals first; or the Board of Trustees may have to approve proposals.)

Eighty per cent reported that their institutions had such formal or informal controls in addition to the peer review committee. (We have only uncoded data on these additional controls. Many, perhaps most, of the ones mentioned are formal.)

THE EFFICACY OF PEER GROUP REVIEW

Now that we have described the structure of peer group review as it presently operates, now that we have seen some of the ways in which committees make their decisions, what can we say about the action they have taken thus far? In other words, how efficacious has the system of peer group review been in its present and actual form?

Efficacy is, of course, a hard concept to define and measure in any field of human action. Our National Survey data provide four ways of approaching efficacy, although none is to be taken as a final or absolute measure of what we are trying to understand.

The first approach is through the respondents' reports about the actual practices of the peer review committees, that is, about their actual decisions to approve, request revision, or reject the research protocols that were submitted to them. Certainly, the record of committees' performances indicates their efficacy in some sense. However, we shall have to qualify the meaning of this indicator, presently, when we discuss it in more detail.

Our second approach is based upon what our respondents told us in answer to the following direct question about committee effectiveness:

> How effective, would you say, is the operation of your institutional review committee in helping to protect the rights and welfare of the human subjects of clinical research in your institution? (Check only *one*)
>
> a. Very effective
> b. Effective to a degree
> c. Ineffective because it has little power
> d. Much of the clinical research that is done does not get submitted to the committee for review
> e. Other (please specify)

Our third approach involves use of an index of strictness (permissiveness) of an institution's review committee with respect to requiring that the risks of proposed research for its human subjects are counterbalanced by the potential benefit to them, to others, or to medical science. The issue of informed voluntary consent is also included, but in a minor way. This index is based on our respondents' estimates of the decisions their institutional review committees would make in their review of the last three hypothetical research proposals presented in our questionnaire. This index is analogous in construction to the "permissiveness index" described in our discussion of expressed ethical standards in Chapter 4;[21] the only difference is that that index involved respondents' reports of *their own* decisions regarding the last three hypothetical proposals, whereas this one involves their estimates of *their committees'* decisions. The assumption in this approach is that the strictness of a committee's ethical standards must be one determinant of its efficacy as a social control mechanism with respect to the protection of the human subjects of biomedical research.

Finally, the fourth approach relating to committee efficacy is the most indirect. We asked our respondents in the following question how they thought the work of the committee had been received by the researchers in their institution who were subject to having their proposals reviewed by the committee:

> Generally speaking, would you say that the work of the institutional review committee *with respect to its review of the ethical aspects of clinical research* has been well received by the clinical researchers in your institution? Please do not include as opposition such things as the common complaint about increased paperwork.
>
> a. Very well received
> b. Fairly well received, no opposition
> c. Some opposition to the work of the committee
> d. Much opposition to the work of the committee
> e. Other (please specify)

We mentioned earlier that none of these four indicators should be taken as a final or absolute measure of the efficacy of the peer review process. Let us amplify that statement.

First, all four of the indicators depend completely on the knowledge and veracity of just one respondent per institution. The replies constituting the indicators, "reported committee effectiveness," "strictness of committee ethical standards," and "reception of the work of the committee" required rather difficult, accurate perceptions, evaluations, and probably aggregation by respondents of intangible properties of the review committees and of

---

[21] See footnote 22, Chapter 4, infra.

clinical researchers in their institutions. Moreover, the probability that there was some tendency on the part of respondents to report favorably about their institutions with respect to the efficacy of their peer review procedures should be kept in mind when examining the data.

Secondly, contrary to what might be expected, there is little or no empirical intercorrelation among "record of committee actions regarding review of protocols," "reported committee effectiveness," and "strictness of committee ethical standards." Also, as will be seen, all four indicators tend to have different review-involved structural correlates. These findings suggest that the indicators may be tapping different, at least partly independent, dimensions of efficacy, or that one (or more) of them serves better as an indicator than the other(s).

These then are problems concerning our indicators of efficacy. However, it should be remembered that despite these limitations: (1) the findings we are about to present represent the first systematic exploration of the question of peer review committee efficacy based upon empirical data from a national sample; and (2) the great majority of the respondents in the National Survey were in positions in their institutions which should have made them knowledgeable even with respect to the intangible properties we are concerned with here. Eighty-seven per cent of them were members of their institutions' review committees, and the rest, although not committee members, were almost certainly selected by their institutions to complete the questionnaire at least partly because of their knowledge of the operation of the committee in their institutions.

We shall now examine each of these four rough measures of efficacy, one at a time. For each we shall present the frequency distribution, as well as any of the previously discussed review-involved structural conditions which our data actually show to be correlates and which we interpret as likely determinants of peer review efficacy.

When we look at the first indicator, the reports of what institutional review committees have done with research protocols—the actual ethical screening decisions made by the committees—we find the following actions taken. The committees in 31% of the institutions, we were told, had required researchers to *revise* their proposed clinical research for ethical reasons in one or more cases, but had made *no rejections*. In 32% of the institutions we were informed that the committee had rejected one or more protocols. Three per cent of the institutions admitted that, although there had been no revisions or rejections of proposals by their committees, there were "one or more instances where an investigator withdrew his proposal when he sensed that revision or rejection for ethical reasons was likely." (In all, 19% of the institutions reported such withdrawals of protocols.) The remaining 34% of the respondents claimed that their committees had required no revisions of protocols submitted to them, made no rejections, and occasioned no withdrawals.

With respect to *rates* of revision, rejection, and withdrawal, 16% of the institutional respondents estimated that their committees had required revision of more than 10% of the proposals reviewed by them; 15% that their committees had rejected more than 3% of the proposals they received; and 9% that more than 1% of the proposals coming before their committees had been withdrawn by investigators to avoid rejection or revision. We have constructed an index or composite rate for each institutional review committee from these particular rates so that what we shall call a "relatively high rate of revision, rejection and/or withdrawal" applies to any committee reported to have required revision of more than 10% of the proposals submitted to it *or* rejected more than 3% of them *or* occasioned withdrawal of more than 1%, *or* acted in any combination of these ways. According to this index, 29% of the committees had a relatively high rate of revision, rejection, and/or withdrawal.

Incidentally, there seems to be some connection between ethical deficiency and scientific deficiency. We asked our respondents whether a protocol that was "rejected or needing modification on ethical grounds generally also lacks merit on purely scientific grounds." Twenty-seven per cent of the respondents said that the committee did generally find that ethically defective proposals also lacked "merit on substantive scientific grounds." Twenty-two per cent said they also lacked "merit on methodological grounds."

The fact that negative action regarding one or more proposals has been effected by peer review committees in 66% of the institutions and that there has been a relatively high rate of negative actions by committees in 29% of the institutions certainly indicates that the committee has had *some degree of efficacy* as a control mechanism in improving the ethical quality of biomedical research using human subjects. However, logical and empirical analysis of this indicator suggests that perhaps often a relatively high rate of revision, rejection, and/or withdrawal is also a sign of something else.

Logically, a higher rate of negative actions by a peer review committee could indicate not only (1) greater effectiveness or strictness of committee operation, but also (2) more frequent production by researchers of proposals which are ethically deficient, or (3) greater inadequacy of "first-line" professional controls, namely, selective recruitment, socialization, and other formal and informal colleague controls, or (4) any combination of these three situations. For example, a 5% rejection rate (relatively high) by a review committee would result in an institution where other formal and informal controls are poor and where comparatively many ethically deficient proposals are produced by researchers, but where the committee is relatively permissive and ineffective, so that out of the 100 protocols it reviews, it rejects only 5 of the 10 which a more effective and stricter committee would have rejected. But a 5% rejection rate would also result in another institution where only .5 proposals are ethically deficient out of the 100 which are produced, get through other informal and formal colleague controls, and are submitted to the committee, which is very strict and effective and rejects all 5.

Moreover, as we have already mentioned, our data show little or no relationship between reported rate of revision, rejection, and/or withdrawal and either estimated effectiveness of a committee (our second indicator of efficacy) or the strictness of a committee's ethical standards (our third indicator of efficacy). The same proportion, 29%, both of committees judged to be "very effective" ($N = 200$) as well as of those characterized as "less than very effective" ($N = 62$) were found to have a relatively high rate of revision, rejection, and/or withdrawal. And 25% of relatively permissive committees ($N = 72$), 30% of less permissive committees ($N = 74$), and 34% of strict ones ($N = 80$) reported relatively high rate of negative actions. (Although it is in the expected direction, a percentage difference of 9% is relatively small).

On the basis of the preceding analysis then, one could conclude that often, possibly more often than not, a higher rate of negative actions by a peer review committee signaled a higher incidence of ethically deficient proposals and/or the more frequent inadequacy of "first-line" professional controls rather than, or in addition to, greater effectiveness or strictness of committee operation. However, considering the problems (already seen and to be seen) with the measures of "reported committee effectiveness" and "strictness of committee ethical standards" used in the analysis, we have some reservation about this conclusion. What *can* be said more definitely is that records and rates of committee actions regarding review of protocols can be used to indicate committee efficacy in the sense that a committee exercised its social control function on behalf of the human subjects of biomedical research comparatively frequently or, at least, sometimes; however, *not* in the sense that it exercised that function as frequently or as well as it could or should have.

Since the committees varied in their rates of revision, rejection, and/or withdrawal, we tried to discover any review-involved structural determinant of this variation. We found one correlate that lends itself to such an interpretation. Review committees whose decision processes included a formal appeal procedure were more likely to have a relatively high rate of negative action. The committees in 37% of the institutions which had a formal appeal procedure ($N = 117$) also had a relatively high rate of revision, rejection, and/or withdrawal, whereas this was true in 22% of those which did not ($N = 143$). Supplementing what we said earlier, we suggest that the presence of an appeal procedure may allow committees to feel more free in their ethical criticism of research proposals. Given the existence of a correcting mechanism at the next stage of peer review, they may be more willing to be bolder in their decisions to say "no" to a colleague. Of course, the establishment of a formal appeal mechanism might also be the *consequence* of a high rate of negative actions by an institutional review committee, insofar as this has generated effective pressures from researchers for such a means of appealing committee decisions.

We turn now from the committees' reported record of decisions in reviewing protocols to our second measure of their efficacy. This is the indicator that uses what our respondents told us in answer to our direct question about the committee's effectiveness. Seventy-six per cent responded that they thought their committees were "very effective." The others, of course, chose one of the lesser degrees of effectiveness—22% indicated their committee was "effective to a degree," while only 2% (6 institutions) admitted that it was "ineffective because it has little power" or that "much of the clinical research that is actually done does not get submitted to the committee for review."

As to review-involved structural correlates, our respondents tended to see their committees as more effective when it was committee policy to review all clinical research conducted by researchers in the institution, when there was a policy of continuing formal review by the committee, and when the committee met as a body after pre-review of proposals. More precisely, 80% of those committees reported to review all clinical research ($N = 246$) were viewed by our respondents as "very effective," as against 55% of those which reviewed only clinical research involving a formal proposal for funds either just from P.H.S. or also from other sources ($N = 42$). Eighty-two per cent of the committees reported to have continuing formal review ($N = 112$) were seen as "very effective," 76% of those where there was continuing review, but either by institutional agents other than the committee or by the committee using more informal procedures ($N = 110$), and 67% of those where there was no continuing review at all ($N = 64$). Finally, 79% of committees reported to meet as a body after pre-review of protocols ($N = 216$) were believed to be "very effective," and 74% of those in which individual members pre-reviewed protocols but often did not meet as a body ($N = 31$), as against 63% of those which met as a body but with no pre-review of protocols by any of the members ($N = 40$).

These three findings may mean that, as intended by the authorities responsible for their establishment, review of all clinical research, continuing review, and pre-review before meeting as a body have contributed to the effectiveness of committees in their task of protecting the rights and welfare of the human subjects of biomedical investigations. However, if many of the respondents decided that these three conditions constituted good indicators to use in their estimates of committee effectiveness, this could also explain the correlations.

Our third, more indirect approach to appraising the efficacy of peer review committees involved our index of the strictness of the ethical standards of an institution's review committee, based on a respondent's estimates of the decisions which the committee in his institution would have made in reviewing each of the last three hypothetical proposals presented in the National Survey questionnaire.[22] Using this index, we found that 36% of the committees were characterized as strict, the rest being permissive to a lesser or greater degree. We also found two review-involved structural correlates of committee strictness.

The first finding suggests that use of specialized subcommittees by an institutional review committee contributes to greater strictness of review. For whereas 55% of institutional review committees which reportedly used subcommittees ($N = 22$) were categorized as having strict ethical standards, this was true of 35% of those which had no specialization into subcommittees ($N = 213$).

The second finding is that, in institutions where the respondents said there were additional controls over research using human subjects beyond the peer review committee, 40% ($N = 197$) of the review committees were classified as ethically strict, as against 20% in the institutions reportedly without such additional controls ($N = 51$). We find it difficult to interpret this relationship, although both a strict committee and additional controls would seem to be indicative of institutional concern with regard to provision of adequate controls over biomedical research using human subjects.

Our fourth, most indirect attempt to evaluate committee efficacy was through our respondents' appraisals of how well the work of the committees had been received by the clinical researchers in their institutions. Many people in the biomedical research community had predicted widespread opposition to the "imposition" of P.H.S. guidelines when they were put into effect in 1966. In fact, as our data show, the work of the peer review committees mandated by these guidelines seems to have been relatively well received. In 52% of the institutions in our sample, our respondents reported that the work of the committee was "very well received" by clinical researchers. In another 37%, the committee was "fairly well received, no opposition." In

---

[22] Committees classified as ethically strict were those which respondents estimated would have refused to approve the proposals, as presented, regardless of probability of important medical discovery and also would have rejected the "pulmonary function" proposal or, at least, approved it only if there were virtually no chance of an increase in post-operative complications.

only 11% of the institutions did our respondents admit "some opposition to the work of the committee" on the part of the clinical researchers; none admitted "much opposition." Assuming that our respondents have more or less accurately estimated the response of their colleagues to the P.H.S. initiated control over their research, what light can our data throw upon this perhaps unexpectedly favorable reception to the operation of a social innovation that some researchers might see as "restrictive"?

First, let us look at what seems to have been one review-involved structural determinant of a very good reception for the committee's work. As has been seen, most (70%) of the institutions in our National Survey reported that they had had a review procedure which scrutinized the ethical aspects of proposed clinical research before the National Institutes of Health required that one be put into effect. In about two-fifths of these institutions having had a preexisting review procedure, the procedure was reported to have met the new requirements of N.I.H. to the degree that no changes had been required by N.I.H. or made by the institution. As might be expected, it was among those institutions which not only had had a review procedure predating the N.I.H. guidelines, but also had neither chosen nor been required to make any revisions in it that the subsequent operation of this procedure was most frequently "very well received" and not opposed by an institution's clinical investigators. Sixty-nine per cent of the respondents from institutions where no revisions in a preexisting procedure had been required by N.I.H. or made by the institution on its own initiative ($N = 68$) said their clinical researchers generally received the work of the committee very well. By contrast, this was true for 51% of the institutions where minor changes had been required by N.I.H. ($N = 49$), for 47% of those which had made some changes on their own ($N = 47$), for 45% of those which had had no previous review procedure ($N = 84$) and, most strikingly, for only 33% of those where N.I.H. had required major revisions in a preexisting procedure ($N = 24$).

Second, what seems to have been another determinant of the acceptance of peer review by biomedical researchers who are involved in studies using human subjects is the rate of revision, rejection, and/or withdrawal resulting from peer review. Where review committees had a relatively high rate of negative actions, their work was much less likely to be viewed favorably and without opposition by an institution's clinical researchers. Thirty-seven per cent of the institutions with committees having a relatively high rate of revision, rejection, and/or withdrawal ($N = 75$) reported that the work of those committees was very well received by their clinical investigators, as against 58% of those institutions with committees having a lower rate ($N = 182$). Thus, it seems fairly clear that another reason the amount of opposition to this social innovation, the peer review committee, was as small as it was on the part of the people most directly affected by it (the clinical researchers) was because, as we have seen, over 70% of the committees which were set up have a low rate of negative actions, including over a third which have never done anything but approve the research proposals that were submitted.

However, we should not too quickly conclude that this finding of a relationship between "rate of revision, rejection, and/or withdrawal as a result of peer review," our first indicator of committee efficacy, and this fourth indicator of efficacy means that opposition to peer review materialized more often when the committee most fully complied with the P.H.S. mandate and that this restrictive social innovation was accepted so favorably because its restrictiveness was somewhat tempered by the receiving social institution. For, as we have shown, "rate of revision, rejection, and/or withdrawal" is essentially not related either to "reported committee effectiveness" (our second measure of efficacy) or to "strictness of committee ethical standards" (our third measure). In addition, both of these latter measures are found to be related to "reception of the work of the committee by the clinical researchers in an institution" *in the opposite direction* from that in which "rate of revision, rejection, and/or withdrawal" is related to it. That is, the *more effective* and the *more strict* the committee, the *more likely* it was very well received.

Finally, two findings concerning other review-involved structural correlates of very good reception of the committee add to the previous point. First our data show that in institutions which required that all clinical research be reviewed by the committee, the work of the committee was more likely to have been "very well received." Fifty-five per cent of the respondents who said that the committee in their institution reviewed all clinical investigations ($N = 240$) also thought that the committee was very well received by the institution's clinical researchers, whereas 38% of those from institutions where the committee reviewed less than all clinical research ($N = 42$) thought the committee received such a favorable reception. This seems to indicate that though researchers may prefer less rather than more restrictions on their work, once restrictions have been imposed they react more favorably when local institutional policy, restrictive or not, is applied universalistically. The finding seems to imply that researchers think it more fair if no researcher is exempt from peer review just because his research is funded by some other agency than P.H.S.

Second, we find a relationship in institutions between the proportion of review committee members required for approval of proposed clinical research and the reception of the work of the committee by the institution's clinical investigators. The most favorable reception was found at institutions where unanimity of committee members was required for approval; the least favorable, where no proportion was stipulated. More specifically, 66% of institutions where unanimity of the committee members voting on a proposal was said to be required (113) reported that their clinical researchers had received the committee's work very well, in comparison to 54% of institutions where a two-thirds majority was required (13), 44% of those where a simple majority was required (72), and 37% of those where no specific proportion was stipulated (75). Once again, although researchers may generally dislike restrictions on their work, this finding seems to indicate another specifying condition. Perhaps, even though a requirement of unanimity could make approval of their protocols by the committee somewhat more difficult, researchers prefer this to the legal and professional vulnerability or the lingering doubts which less than unanimous approval by peers may leave.[23] This interpretation is even more plausible considering that, as has been mentioned, unanimity in important decision-making pertaining to shared fundamental values is more in accord with professional collegiality.

Thus, these several findings suggest that by no means does fuller institutional regulation of the ethical aspects of biomedical research using human subjects necessarily lead to greater opposition by clinical investigators, but rather that the type of control and other variable conditions must be specified if researcher reaction is to be correctly understood and anticipated.

In conclusion, reviewing all the evidence we have presented about the efficacy of peer review committees, what can we say? Certainly the majority of the committees have shown at least some efficacy in their assigned task of safeguarding the welfare and rights of the human subjects of biomedical research, regardless of which of the four approaches to appraising efficacy one looks at. Undoubtedly, because of the peer review group mode of social control, ethical practices in this area are much better than they were in the early 1960's and before. However, using these measures, we also see causes for concern in at least a significant minority of institutions.[24] Moreover, the

---

[23] Such concerns of researchers may also partly account for the preceding finding that researchers more frequently received the work of the committee most favorably when it reviewed all clinical research without exception.

[24] It should be added here that, using our National Survey data, we can compare members of biomedical research institutions who serve on their peer review committees with those who do not, in regard to the strictness of their expressed ethical standards as measured by our permissiveness index. Since, as discussed earlier, the National Survey sample is biased toward senior people and review committee members—one per institution—who were chosen as institutional respondents for our study, the findings are presented as only suggestive: approximately the same proportion of those respondents who were review committee members and of those who were not are classified as relatively permissive—32% of those who were committee members (216) as compared with 30% of those who were not (37); however, only 37% of those who were committee members were strict as against 54% of those who were not committee members. When we control

data from our Intensive Two-Institution Study reinforce this concern. It is apparently the policy in both of the institutions we studied for all research on humans to be reviewed by the appropriate committee, yet 8% of the researchers interviewed volunteered, without being asked, that one or more of their biomedical studies involving human subjects had not been reviewed. In addition, as Chapter 3 has shown, according to our two Risk-Benefit Ratios based on the interviewees' own estimates, as high as 18% of the studies still being done in these two institutions have been classified as less favorable for the human subjects involved, and 8% have been categorized as least favorable, that is, involving risks which at least approach being in excess of benefit for the subjects concerned, for others, and for medical science. Thus, if the data from our two studies are called in evidence, there is serious need for improvement in both the structure and procedures of the N.I.H.-mandated review committees.

On the basis of our National Survey, we have seen that there do seem to be structural determinants of greater or lesser efficacy of such committees, although different ones depending on which approach to determining efficacy one uses. As such determinants and indicators of efficacy are clarified, further specified, and validated, they should become useful guides to policy for constructing improved review committees.

---

by whether respondents were clinical researchers or physicians, on the one hand, or laymen, on the other, these findings remain essentially unchanged. Considering the serious obligations of peer review committees with respect to the protection of the welfare and rights of the human subjects of biomedical research, those selected to serve on them should be of the highest ethical standards. Findings that committee members are, in fact, less frequently ethically strict and no less frequently permissive as reviewers than are others in their institutions, must be, if in any way representative, matters for concern.

10

SOCIAL CONTROL: HAVE MEDICAL SCHOOLS BEEN ETHICAL LEADERS?

As we saw in our sketch of the evolution of peer review, the impetus to the reform of standards and practices in the use of human subjects in biomedical research has tended to come in much greater measure from governmental response to public outcry, a response showing itself in F.D.A. and N.I.H. regulation, than directly from the medical profession at large or biomedical research profession itself. There have, of course, been a few distinguished individual exceptions. For example, in addition to the effects of governmental regulation, some weight in pushing forward reforms in the use of human subjects has come from a few individual medical researchers such as Dr. Henry Beecher in the United States and Dr. M. Pappworth in England. We have also seen, in our chapter on ethical socialization, that the medical profession has hardly been an innovator in that mode of social control. Is it indeed the case that the profession has been laggard in proposing new agencies of social control, in using new structures and processes for adequately realizing the value of humane therapy that it so proudly proclaims on all appropriate occasions? To answer this question, in this chapter we examine in considerable detail the performance of the medical schools in comparison to other types of biomedical research institutions and conclude that they unfortunately have not been ethical leaders with regard to peer group review. They have a proud record of *scientific* leadership, but their record in *ethical* innovation is not distinguished.

In *The Student Physician* Robert K. Merton states:

> . . . Medical schools [are] the guardians of the values basic to the effective practice of medicine.
> . . . It is their function to transmit the culture of medicine and to advance that culture. It is their task to shape the novice into the effective practitioner of medicine, to give him the best available knowledge and skills, and to provide him with a professional identity so that he comes to think, act, and feel like a physician.[1]

---

[1] Robert K. Merton, "Some Preliminaries to a Sociology of Medical Education," Robert K. Merton, George G. Reader, and Patricia L. Kendall, eds., in *The Student Physician* (Cambridge, Mass.: Harvard University Press, 1957), p. 7.

That is, medical schools are the agencies officially claiming and actually having prime responsibility for the education and training of those who will carry on the medical profession as practitioners, as researchers, and as teachers. In the United States Abraham Flexner left, through the medium of his monumental report, a legacy of ideals of professional excellence for the medical school. Three World Conferences on Medical Education and numerous authoritative voices in the profession have called medical schools to their mission of continuing and adaptive attainment of these ideals. Thus, the proclaimed obligations of their function constrain medical schools to be, or at least to strive to be, leaders in the profession with regard to skills, technology, and scholarship, on the one hand, and in the observance of professional ethics, on the other. They are expected to be the natural environment of role models for the profession, especially for its new recruits, in all these areas.

The ethics of experimentation on human beings, from their intimation in the Hippocratic Oath to their more recent elaboration in codes, such as the Declaration of Helsinki, have been very much a part of the medical tradition, related to that concern for the good of the individual which is entrusted to the physician. Medical schools, then, if they are to be the ethical leaders that the ideals of the profession would make them, should be in the forefront of efforts to safeguard the rights and welfare of the human subjects of biomedical research.

Now, using data collected largely in our National Survey, we present a comparison of medical schools with other types of biomedical research institutions. This comparison will indicate that medical schools are far from having been leaders in providing social controls, especially those of formal peer review, to protect the subjects of biomedical human experimentation.

In the previous chapter we presented findings that drew a picture of the structure, functioning, and efficacy of those committees entrusted with peer review of clinical research in all biomedical research institutions in the United States. A number of structural conditions that might reasonably be expected to contribute to the efficacy of such formal review of clinical research, and commonly instituted for just that purpose, were found to correlate with one or another of the four indicators of committee efficacy used. To make the comparisons we need of medical schools and other institutions, we shall examine the variation of the occurrence of each of these several indicators and conditions (as well as three additional conditions mandated, recommended, or suggested by P.H.S.)[2] in different types of institutions. These are medi-

---

[2] These additional conditions are: early submission of formal assurance of compliance with P.H.S. policy, review of all clinical research proposals for P.H.S. funds prior to their submission to P.H.S., and inclusion of one or more "outsiders" as peer review committee members.

cal schools, teaching hospitals affiliated with medical schools, mental hospitals, and what we have called "other institutions," that is, a residual category that includes teaching hospitals not fully affiliated with medical schools, general hospitals, and other institutions where biomedical experimentation using human subjects is conducted.

The distinction we make between a "medical school" and a "teaching hospital affiliated with a medical school" is based on whether or not a teaching hospital affiliated with a particular medical school has submitted its own assurance of compliance with peer review requirements to P.H.S., that is, in effect, whether or not it has its own institutional peer review committee separate from and at least relatively autonomous of any peer review committee the medical school has. When teaching hospitals affiliated with medical schools have their own peer review apparatus and consequently have completed a separate questionnaire for us, we classify them as "teaching hospitals affiliated with medical schools." Those institutions we call "medical schools" have responded for themselves and, at least sometimes, for teaching hospitals included under the assurances they submitted to P.H.S. Later this distinction will be seen to have implications for our analysis.

When we do examine the differential occurrence, in medical schools as compared to the other types of institutions, of the aforementioned conditions and indicators regarding peer review which are desirable for the better protection of human subjects, the findings are those presented in Tables 10.1, 10.2, and 10.3, which form the basis of our analysis in this chapter.

As inspection shows, in regard to none of the aspects of peer review considered in Table 10.1 can medical schools be construed to be leaders. On the contrary, in comparison to institutions of other kinds, especially mental hospitals and "other institutions" (we shall shortly discuss the special case of teaching hospitals affiliated with medical schools), medical schools had the lowest frequency, by a notable margin, in every aspect considered— namely, having had a review procedure before the P.H.S. required one; if an institution had a prior review procedure, having had no major changes in it required by P.H.S.; having a committee which reviewed *all* clinical research; having a committee which reviewed all clinical research proposals for P.H.S. funds *before* their submission to P.H.S.; having a committee which included one or more "outsiders" (that is, clinical research specialists or physicians from other institutions or persons who have nonmedical roles in the larger community and are not members of the institution) as regular members; and having had the work of the committee very well received by the institution's clinical investigators.

Using some of our other data, we tried to explain these findings by controlling for possible explanatory factors. For example, our other data show that medical schools, in comparison to other types of institutions, more often

Table 10.1. Conditions and Indicator Regarding Peer Review Which Are in Accord with Better Protection of Human Subjects by Type of Institution

	Medical Schools	Teaching Hospitals Affiliated with Med. Schools	Mental Hospitals	Other Institutions
a. Institution had review procedure before P.H.S. required one.	51% (57)	68% (57)	80% (88)	75% (84)
b. If institution had a prior procedure, no major changes were required by P.H.S.	65% (29)	92% (38)	90% (68)	93% (59)
c. Committee reviewed all clinical research.	74% (58)	93% (57)	88% (93)	84% (83)
d. All clinical research proposals for P.H.S. funds were peer reviewed before submission to P.H.S.	50% (58)	55% (56)	84% (89)	74% (80)
e. Committee had one or more "outsiders" as regular members.	9% (55)	17% (48)	27% (84)	28% (72)
f. Work of committee was very well received by clinical researchers.	33% (57)	46% (57)	58% (89)	63% (79)

tended to turn out a relatively high number of papers per clinical investigator. "Number of papers published per clinical researcher" might be considered a rough indicator of the science orientation in an institution. However, when we controlled by this variable and by other relevant variables in the above findings, none clearly proved to interpret any of those findings. However, N's in these three-variable tables tended to be relatively small.[3]

---

[3] It should be stressed that our purpose here was exclusively to look in our data for any factors which would help to "interpret" the findings in question. As we have reported, we found none of these. However, we did discover that—with respect to in-

We have to go beyond these data to suggest a possible and partial explanation of the lagging of medical schools behind other kinds of biomedical research institutions in the introduction and effective use of peer group review. Our explanation lies in the *professional* character of biomedical researchers. Although there is still much that is unsettled in this field, the sociology of the professions has come to agree on the centrality of the values of autonomy and self-regulation for all professions.[4] Both the medical profession at large and the biomedical research profession in particular make strong claims to autonomy and self-regulation on the grounds that only they have the sufficient knowledge, skill, and moral trustworthiness to judge and regulate the performance of all their members. The values and associated beliefs or ideologies that physicians in practice or in research hold are that self-regulation can be most effectively achieved through the application of high standards for recruitment and training from medical school on and through the "normal" operation of colleague controls in teaching, practice, and research. Moreover, it is also a strongly held value in the medical profession that, as far as possible, controls should be *informal* colleague controls. Such controls are much preferred to either local-institution or professional *formal* controls. Formal controls are seen as unnecessarily restrictive and involving bureaucratic red tape and distant authorities who are not as competent to judge an individual professional's work as are his local peers.[5] Attempts at control by agencies outside of the profession are seen as worst

---

dividual findings, although not consistently for the whole set of findings—the control variables used did "specify" circumstances under which the original relationships were more and less pronounced. But these are beyond the scope of the present discussion. Regarding our usage here of the terms "interpret" and "specify," see Herbert Hyman, *Survey Design and Analysis* (Glencoe, Ill.: The Free Press, 1955), Chapter 7.

[4] For a general statement, see Bernard Barber, "Some Problems in the Sociology of the Professions," in Kenneth S. Lynn, ed., *The Professions in America* (Boston, Mass.: Houghton Mifflin, 1965). For an early and very influential statement, see E. M. Carr-Saunders and P. A. Wilson, *The Professions* (Cambridge, England: The Clarendon Press, 1936). Talcott Parsons' many essays in this field have been important both for their sociological analysis in general and for their specific application to medicine. See, for example, his "Some Theoretical Considerations Bearing on the Field of Medical Sociology," in Parsons, *Social Structure and Personality* (New York: The Free Press of Glencoe, 1964). Finally, for a very specific and empirically based discussion of these problems in the medical profession at large, see Eliot Freidson, *Profession of Medicine* (New York: Dodd, Mead, 1970), Chapters 7, 8, esp. pp. 137, 161–162.

[5] For some empirical evidence on this point, see Walter J. McNerney, et al., *Hospital and Medical Economics*, 2 vols. (Chicago: Hospital Research and Educational Trust, 1962), p. 1325. McNerney, on the basis of his study of the voluntary health system in Michigan, indicates that formal controls are perceived by physicians as encroachments on professional independence to make decisions.

of all; hence the great resistance to suggested control by local communities, social service agencies, or state or federal governments.[6] We are now, of course, only reporting what values are asserted; we are not assessing the scientific validity of these claims and statements. It is probably the case that *both* formal and informal modes of social control have *both* functions and dysfunctions for the effective performance of practice and research.[7] We are now only trying to suggest that the greater valuation of informal controls would lead to a certain resistance to accept formal peer group review, especially when it is mandated by a federal agency.

It has been stated by a close student of these matters that "medical schools are the guardians of the values basic to the effective practice of medicine." Of course, they are also, at the present time, the principal centers for biomedical research. In our chapter on socialization we saw that they seem to be more effective at the present time in socializing their students who become clinical investigators into the value of research than into the ethics of the use of human subjects in the research that is so highly valued. And because the formal peer group review procedures that are required by N.I.H. do in fact limit in some measure existing levels of professional autonomy and self-regulation with regard to research, it would seem to follow that the medical school clinical research community would accept this innovation less willingly than other types of institutions where the "value of research" was less strongly established. Such outside formal control is felt to infringe upon the basic values and interests of the medical school research community. Given such values, this community would be, and our data show it in fact is, more resistant to formal peer group review.

We now turn to several of our findings to show how they lend support to the explanation we have just given for the laggard pattern of the medical schools. Perhaps the finding from our National Survey data that there was a considerably poorer reception of and more opposition to the work of the peer review committee among clinical investigators in medical schools than in other types of institutions (Table 10.1f) constitutes the best corroboration for the preceding interpretation. However, it should be noted that this opposition was on the part of only the clinical investigators in an institution. But more, or at least equally, crucial to the kind of resistance to formal peer review which could have effected the differences between medical schools and other types of institutions reported in Table 10.1, *a* through *e*, would

---

[6] See any one of many statements by the A.M.A. Or, more specifically, see the report of a speech by Dr. Walter C. Bornemeier, then President of the A.M.A., concerning the need for control of proposed neighborhood medical clinics by the profession rather than by lay agencies. *New York Times*, Nov. 30, 1970, p. 28.

[7] For empirical evidence that informal colleague controls do not work very well in the practice of medicine, see Freidson, *op. cit.*, Chap. 7.

have been those advocates and supporters of clinical research who had weighty, direct or indirect influence upon institutional policy making, such as administrators, prestigious physicians, and so on, who very frequently number nonresearchers among their ranks. Moreover, the opposition suggested in Table 10.1*f* was with respect to the actual work and implementation of peer review which had already been carried out by an institution's committee; this is analytically distinguishable from original and continuing opposition to peer review as a matter of principle.

Data from our Intensive Two-Institution Study at University Hospital and Research Center (a medical school complex) and at Community and Teaching Hospital, which falls into the "other institutions" category, give further support to our interpretation. Seventeen per cent of the clinical investigators interviewed at University Hospital and Research Center ($N = 322$) felt that the P.H.S. policy generally requiring "voluntary informed consent" from an individual before he may be accepted as a research subject was restrictive; at Community and Teaching Hospital only 7% of the clinical researchers ($N = 55$) felt this way. Moreover, 33% of the clinical researchers at University Hospital and Research Center ($N = 320$) opposed the inclusion of "qualified layman (such as lawyers)" on peer review committees, whereas 15% of those at Community and Teaching Hospital ($N = 54$) expressed opposition to such "outsiders."[8]

It may have been noticed that in Table 10.1, *a* through *f*, the frequencies of teaching hospitals affiliated with medical schools were most often in an ordinal position between those of medical schools, on the one hand, and those of mental hospitals and "other institutions," on the other (Table 10.1, *a*, *d*, *e*, and *f*). However, in two cases these teaching hospitals affiliated with medical schools are found to be much closer to mental hospitals and "other institutions" than to medical schools (Table 10.1, *b* and *c*). These observations suggest that, although by their nature teaching hospitals affiliated with medical schools participate in the professional ethos of medical schools and are involved in their structure more than any other type of institution, nevertheless, they are also to some extent *structurally and culturally* independent of and different from medical schools and thus might have different responses to social control innovations.[9] In support of this point, it should be recalled that earlier we explained that the teaching hospi-

---

[8] Insofar as in our Two-Institution Study we guaranteed respondents anonymity and assured them we would, as best possible, also try to prevent identification of their institutions, we believe it is in accordance with these assurances to withhold presentation of the comparison between University Hospital and Research Center and Community and Teaching Hospital on the variables in Table 10.1.

[9] The above discussed controls (by "papers published per clinical investigator," and other relevant variables) made regarding the findings presented in Table 10.1 did not

tals included in this category have sent P.H.S. their own, separate assurances of compliance and have their own peer review committees at least partly independent of the committees for their medical schools. This is in contrast to other teaching hospitals which are less independent of the medical schools with which they are affiliated in that they have not submitted their own assurances of compliance to N.I.H. and are included under the peer review apparatus of their medical schools. In addition, on the one hand, many members of such teaching hospitals also hold teaching or research positions in the medical schools with which their hospitals are affiliated, and hence are at least partly involved in the medical school subculture. But on the other hand, some hospitals become affiliated with medical schools only later in their histories, after they have developed a "non-medical school" character and tradition; also sometimes teaching hospitals affiliated with medical schools are geographically separated from the medical schools with which they are affiliated, so that the cultural and social influence of the latter upon them is diminished.

Thus, the combination of similarities and differences found in Table 10.1, *a* through *f*, between medical schools and teaching hospitals affiliated with medical schools not only is seen to make sense, but also can be construed to support the interpretation suggested as to why medical schools were not found to have been the ethical leaders they are expected to be.

We turn now to further findings comparing medical schools and other types of institutions in respect of other conditions and indicators regarding peer review which are favorable for better protection of human subjects. Looking at the indicators and conditions in Table 10.2, we find essentially no consistent significant differences between medical schools and other kinds of institutions. However, not being different again shows lack of leadership. We suggest that this similarity of medical schools and other institutions is the result of either one of two situations. Either there are other values or interests in medical schools which counter the resistance to peer review engendered by the autonomy and self-regulation components of their professional ethos, although not enough to have made them leaders in whichever aspect of peer review is in question. Or the item of peer review in question was felt to infringe little upon professional autonomy. In Table 10.3 we see two cases in which medical schools, in comparison especially to mental hospitals and "other institutions," had the highest frequency by a notable margin. But, when looked at more closely, in one of these cases this apparent leadership can be shown to be probably spurious and, in the other, it can be seen to be "the exception which proves the rule."

---

interpret the unique position of teaching hospitals affiliated with medical schools in the findings.

Table 10.2. Other Indicators and Conditions Regarding Peer Review Which Are in Accord with Better Protection of Human Subjects by Type of Institution

	Medical Schools	Teaching Hospitals Affiliated with Med. Schools	Mental Hospitals	Other Institutions
a. Committee was reported to be very effective.	68% (57)	80% (57)	82% (91)	72% (83)
b. Committee had strict ethical standards.	28% (50)	42% (50)	30% (77)	44% (73)
c. Committee met as a body after pre-review.	69% (58)	77% (57)	76% (92)	77% (83)
d. Institution had some kind of continuing review.	78% (58)	77% (56)	77% (93)	77% (82)
e. Institution had controls in addition to committee.	81% (58)	82% (56)	77% (92)	80% (83)
f. Institution had formal appeal procedure.	50% (58)	46% (57)	43% (90)	47% (78)
g. Committee used specialized subcommittees.	14% (56)	11% (53)	7% (87)	8% (75)
h. Unanimity of committee members was required for approval of proposals.	50% (56)	32% (54)	41% (90)	43% (81)

In other words, when all the evidence is considered, the data still indicate that medical schools have not been ethical leaders in respect to efforts to safeguard the rights and welfare of the human subjects of biomedical research. And the hypothesis we have proposed in at least partial interpretation of this situation remains cogent. We now proceed to a more detailed examination of the tables.

In Table 10.2, *a*, *b*, and *c*, medical schools, relative to other types of institutions, are shown to have had the lowest frequency with regard to having a peer review committee reported to be very effective, having a committee characterized by strict ethical standards, and having a committee which met as a body after pre-review of protocols. However, the margins by which they were lowest are not consistently notable enough to justify the placement of any one of these tables in Table 10.1.

In Table 10.2, *d* through *h*—with regard to having some kind of continuing review, having controls in addition to the peer review committee, having a formal appeal procedure, having a committee which used specialized subcommittees, and having a requirement of unanimity of committee members for approval of proposals—the frequencies of medical schools either match those of the other types of institutions, or they exceed them, although either not sufficiently or not consistently enough to legitimately call them leaders in these particular conditions. At least partial explanations for these cases in which medical schools match or slightly surpass other institutions are found, in some cases, in other values and interests in medical schools which probably served to countervail the resistance to peer review fostered by the strong autonomy elements in their professional ethos; and, in the other cases, the conditions of peer review are probably perceived to encroach on professional autonomy relatively little. Taking each of the cases in order, we suggest that these values, interests, and conditions were as follows.

A continuing review (Table 10.2*d*) is the only condition listed in either Table 10.1 or Table 10.2 which was *specifically mandated* by P.H.S. at the time of our National Survey.[10] The other conditions may have been deemed desirable or were recommended, but were not explicitly or strictly required by P.H.S. Therefore, with respect to having a continuing review, the interests of medical schools concerning P.H.S. funding of their clinical research would have been more likely to offset resistance based on their values and beliefs concerning professional autonomy and self-regulation. For, as the main centers for biomedical research in the nation, medical schools had the most to lose in terms of the large amount of clinical research funds coming from P.H.S., both actually and potentially. And, whereas recommendations and implicit intents concerning peer review might safely have been ignored or temporized, an explicit mandate from P.H.S. could not have been.

Having institutional controls other than peer review over the ethical

---

[10] It should be noted that the P.H.S. Regulation, "Protection of the Individual as a Research Subject" (P.H.S. pamphlet, May 1, 1969), which included this mandate was not officially circulated until after the majority of our questionnaires had come in. However, this mandate had been proposed earlier and institutions should have been aware of it. This seems to have been less true with respect to the requirement, also newly published in the same P.H.S. regulation, that all clinical research proposals for P.H.S. funds should be peer reviewed before submission to P.H.S. Moreover, this requirement of review "prior to submission" to P.H.S. was not absolute, allowing "whenever possible," or review "prior to issuance of the award," when not possible.

aspects of clinical research (Table 10.2*e*) is presumably a condition more in accord with medical values and ideology than a formal review procedure required by an agency outside the profession. For, as defined in our questionnaire, "other institutional controls" included medically preferred informal colleague controls as well as the more traditional formal control of review of proposals by department chairmen. Hence, it is not surprising that medical schools matched other types of institutions in their frequency.

Having a formal procedure by which an investigator can appeal a negative decision of the peer review committee (Table 10.2*f*) obviously constituted an institutional condition as much or more in the interests of clinical research than against those interests, and therefore, would have faced little opposition.

An institution's having a peer review committee which utilized specialized subcommittees (Table 10.2*g*) was, of itself, probably perceived as infringing little upon professional autonomy. Therefore, it was probably resisted relatively little. Moreover, it is a condition which has been shown to be partly a function of the size of an institution's clinical research operation, the largest of which tends to be found in medical schools.

Finally, insofar as medical schools are the guardians of the basic values and beliefs of the profession of medicine, it might be expected that the notion of a professional group, such as a peer review committee, as a company of near-equals sharing essentially a single set of values would be more salient in medical schools than in the other types of research institutions. And, consequently, the tendency to want and require consensus and unanimity in such a group, especially in making decisions about the ethical acceptability of proposed investigations involving the use of human beings as subjects, clearly a matter of great importance to the group's shared basic values, probably would be greater in medical schools than in other institutions. Moreover, the need to deal with the greater volume of clinical research carried on in medical schools might heighten this tendency for peer review committees in medical schools. Therefore, in medical schools this tendency could have countervailed resistance to it stemming from medical school autonomy values and interests, to the degree that medical schools somewhat surpassed the other kinds of institutions in requiring unanimity of committee members for approval of proposals (Table 10.2*h*).

In sum, the several findings in Table 10.2 include no case in which medical schools can clearly be considered to have been leaders regarding peer review, even though they are seen to have matched, more or less, the other types of institutions in the aspects considered. Also, close analysis of these several findings has been found to support our interpretation that resistance based on the strong autonomy elements of the medical school ethos was a determinant of this laggard condition.

Now let us look at our last findings, as presented in Table 10.3. In contrast to what we have seen thus far, Table 10.3 presents two findings in which medical schools seem to have been leaders with regard to peer review.

Table 10.3. Final Indicator and Condition Regarding Peer Review Which Seem in Accord with Better Protection of Human Subjects by Type of Institution

	Medical Schools	Teaching Hospitals Affiliated with Med. Schools	Mental Hospitals	Other Institutions
a. Committee had relatively high rate of revision, rejection, and/or withdrawal of proposals as a result of peer review.	38% (50)	43% (54)	23% (86)	19% (74)
b. Institution gave formal assurance of compliance with P.H.S. policy early (1966).	88% (50)	70% (43)	35% (75)	40% (67)

In the first finding (Table 10.3*a*), medical schools, along with teaching hospitals affiliated with medical schools, are seen to have had a relatively high rate of revision, rejection, and/or withdrawal of clinical research proposals as a result of peer review considerably more often than either mental hospitals or "other institutions." However, as we suggested in the last chapter, such a higher rate of negative action by a peer review committee in an institution may simply have indicated the more frequent production by researchers of proposals which were ethically deficient and/or the greater inadequacy of "first-line" professional controls (namely selective recruitment, socialization, and other formal and informal colleague controls), rather than the greater effectiveness or strictness of committee operation. If this is the case, this finding can be added to those in Table 10.1 as an instance in which medical schools (and teaching hospitals affiliated with medical schools) fell short of being ethical leaders in matters pertaining to the safeguarding of human subjects in biomedical experimentation. But, even if, on the basis of what we said earlier, we cannot be certain that this is the case, this finding is at best ambiguous and cannot safely be used as an instance in which medical schools lead the field in some process of peer review.

In the second finding (Table 10.3*b*), medical schools are seen, clearly and notably more frequently than the other types of institutions, to have given formal assurance. of compliance with the new P.H.S. policy early, that is, in 1966, the year in which it was issued. Submission of this assurance to P.H.S. was required if an institution wanted its investigators to be eligible to continue to receive their share of the large amount of funds for clinical research coming from P.H.S. As the principal centers for such biomedical research, medical schools thus had interests which dictated conformity with this requirement much more urgently than did those of other kinds of institutions. Even though the new P.H.S. policy clashed seriously with the autonomy values and beliefs cherished and promoted by medical schools, considering the dire economic consequences of not submitting an assurance of compliance, there was little choice but to do so.

There is a possible parallel here with the medical schools' conformity with the later P.H.S. requirement of a continuing review. However, there seems to be an important difference which can account for medical schools' notable exceeding of other institutions in frequency of submitting an assurance of compliance in contrast to their mere matching of other institutions in frequency of having a continuing review. Whereas a continuing review was a specific, substantial mechanism required by P.H.S., an assurance of institution-wide compliance involved only "broad guidelines for action" which left implementing mechanisms unspecified, "rather than detailed, substantive regulations."[11] In contrast to establishing a continuing review, there was little effective cost in complying promptly with this particular requirement of submitting a formal assurance; but, as in setting up a continuing review, there was great potential cost in not doing so. It is not surprising, then, that medical schools tended to be quickest in submitting assurances.

Therefore, medical school leadership in this one process of peer review is, upon closer examination, found to have involved an aspect of peer review of little real significance for the protection of human subjects, in comparison with all the other aspects of peer review previously considered. In other words, it is seen to be a kind of "exception that proves the rule" that medical schools have not been ethical leaders regarding peer review.[12]

In summary, the question we have raised in this chapter is "Have medical schools been ethical leaders in the establishment of controls, principally those of formal peer review, for safeguarding the welfare and rights of the

---

[11] Curran, *op. cit.*, p. 578; and Melmon, et al., *op. cit.*, p. 427. The "broad guidelines" were: (a) protection of the rights and welfare of subjects; (b) the obtaining of "informed" consent; and (c) assessment of the risks and potential benefits of the investigation.

[12] It should be noted that controlling the findings in Tables 10.2 and 10.3 by the previously mentioned variables from our data did not interpret this lack of medical school leadership with respect to peer review.

human subjects of biomedical research?" The answer we have found is clearly, "No." The findings with respect to all 16 conditions and indicators regarding peer review and its efficacy which have been examined are impressive. For the "hypothesis" being tested is that medical schools have been leaders, that is, that they are significantly better in performance than the other types of institutions regarding all, or at least most, of the conditions and indicators considered. But as the tables show, in respect to 6 of them the converse of that hypothesis is supported, and in respect to 8 others the null hypothesis is supported. In no case is the hypothesis clearly upheld. In one case of apparent leadership the finding proves to be, at best, ambiguous; and in another, although medical schools are notably higher than other institutions, the condition involved is a relatively unimportant aspect of peer review, making this "the exception that proves the rule."

We have suggested that the autonomy and self-regulation components of the professional ethos, fostered by medical schools which are not only the guardians of the basic values of the medical profession but also the principal centers of biomedical research, have been at least one determinant of the lack of ethical leadership by medical schools in the provision for adequate peer review. These strong values and interests of the medical school, we have argued, have engendered greater resistance to the acceptance and implementation of peer review by the medical school than by other biomedical research institutions.

Perhaps some data from our Two-Institution Study can serve to suggest the possible ethical consequences of the lack of leadership by medical schools in peer review. At University Hospital and Research Center (a medical school complex), 20% of the clinical investigations studied (337) were classified as less favorable according to our Risks-Benefits ratio for Subjects, as against 8% (67) at Community and Teaching Hospital, one of our other institutions type. Even according to our more stringent Risks–All Benefits Ratio, 9% of the investigations examined at University Hospital and Research Center (337) were classified as least favorable in contrast to 2% (67) at Community and Teaching Hospital. Whatever the specific determinants of this situation, the following conclusion suggests itself. Although our data have indicated that all four types of biomedical research institutions are in need of important improvements in their controls meant to protect human subjects, medical schools have been found to be most in need of such improvements. Indeed, these improvements seem to be even more urgent if we remember that medical schools are the prime official agencies of socialization of the medical profession. They have been entrusted with molding those who will be, in the future, the clinical investigators, the physicians attending patients sought after as subjects for clinical research, the members of peer review committees, and the policy makers of the profession regarding such controls. In addition through their example, actions, policies, and ideology, medical schools, which are also the main centers for clinical research, influence the persons presently occupying such major positions in the field of clinical research. In other words, lack of leadership in the controls to safeguard human subjects, a leadership demanded of medical schools by the obligations of their functions, is not only of serious immediate concern, but also seems to augur ill for the future unless significant improvements are made.

1

THE SOCIAL RESPONSIBILITIES OF A POWERFUL PROFESSION: SOME SUGGESTIONS FOR POLICY CHANGE AND REFORM

Having presented all our findings and analysis, we wish to make some suggestions for policy change and reform. From the beginning of our research we have hoped that we could achieve two different but interrelated purposes. First, of course, we hoped to make a contribution to sociological theory and understanding. And second, we hoped that the theory and understanding arrived at through our research would result directly in specific and useful suggestions for policy change and reform. Indeed, the relation between our two purposes has been wholly reciprocal. For not only have theory and findings resulted in suggestions for policy change and reform, but policy questions have, from the beginning, pushed us toward theoretical questions and areas of inquiry that we might not otherwise have seen. For example, our intensive discussion of the efficacy of peer review groups in Chapter 9 was a direct response to the very great policy concern with this matter among governmental and private foundation funding agencies for biomedical research. We must remember that this book has been dealing with a large and ongoing social innovation in which all the interested parties put policy concerns very much to the fore. It was inevitable that we should face those policy concerns quite directly and we have found such confrontation helpful for our theory and analysis, not harmful.

Before proceeding to our specific suggestions for reform, however, it is desirable to put the problems of the biomedical research profession into a larger perspective. For there are definitions of social problems current in our society that include but also transcend the biomedical research profession. These are the definitions and their associated questions about the social responsibilities of any and all powerful professions in our society. If we look first at this larger perspective on the problems of the biomedical research profession, we will be in a better position to offer suggestions for reform that are specific for its needs and problems.

THE SOCIAL RESPONSIBILITIES OF A POWERFUL PROFESSION

We live in a society with enormous and ever-increasing accumulations of knowledge in nearly every sphere of human activity. This knowledge has been produced by the scholarship and science that are a special mark of our society, but some is the product of wise experience as well. And this knowledge, and the technology which often accompanies it, are resources, or as we might otherwise say "power,' for good and evil alike. No wonder that some sociologists think that the phrase, "the knowledge society," characterizes our society as well as any other.

All this powerful knowledge that has been hard-won by the succession of generations must be learned anew and further developed by the expenditure of great energy and intelligence in each generation. Those who put forth such energy and intelligence become "the experts," "the professionals," those who know and know how to use one of the specialized bodies of knowledge without which our kind of society could not be what it is or function as it does. No wonder that some sociologists think that the phrase, "the professional society," characterizes our society as well as any other. We live in a world where scientists, lawyers, the military, biomedical researchers, doctors, economists and a whole set of other professionals, professionalizing groups, and would-be professionals have large amounts of power.[1]

To avoid intended or unintended abuse of the power that knowledge gives, the power must be controlled by appropriate social responsibility. Power is abused when it is used too much on behalf of those who wield it and not enough in the service of those groups in the society, or of the whole society itself, which provide the essential resources and support for its accumulation and exercise. There is an endless tension in all societies between power, wherever it exists, and the social responsibility which guarantees that its use does not become abuse. There is an endless danger, and especially in those situations where it is growing, that power will outrun the capacities of a society to surround it with the necessary mechanisms of social responsibility.[2]

Socially responsible power must be used not just in the interest of those

---

[1] Some have even entered businessmen in this list. For a discussion of that entry, see Bernard Barber, "Is American Business Becoming Professionalized? Analysis of a Social Ideology," in E. A. Tiryakian, ed., *Sociological Theory, Values, and Sociocultural Change: Essays in Honor of Pitirim A. Sorokin* (New York: The Free Press of Glencoe, 1963).

[2] For one case, see Bernard Barber, *Science and the Social Order* (Glencoe, Ill.: The Free Press, 1952), Ch. X, "The Social Control of Science," and especially the sections on "the social consequences of science" and "the social responsibilities of science."

who wield it but in the service of other groups or indeed of the whole society. And this is just what the "professions" claim: that they are in the service of their clients and not of themselves, that the interests and welfare of their clients come first. Where this claim does not exist, where this norm of the direct and overriding importance of the client's interests is not proclaimed, there we do not have "a profession."[3]

To be sure, normative proclamations and actual performance are not the same thing. Some are so cynical that they think of declared norms as "mere window dressing," as cleverly designed concealments for self-interest. And others are so naive and optimistic that they think there never falls a shadow between norm and deed. The sociologist, however, informed both by his theory and by empirical fact, tries first to measure the degree of discrepancy between norm and performance and then goes on to look for some of the several different possible sources of this discrepancy. For the biomedical research profession, that is what we have done in this book. We have found that there is indeed some discrepancy and we have tried to give an account of some of its social sources.

How, then, does a profession become and remain socially responsible? We have already touched upon what is a general problem in this continuing task in which there can only be degrees of success, never perfection. This is the problem of the appropriate mixture of two necessary types of social control in a profession: control from within the profession (internal) and control from outside social structures and processes (external). We now return to this problem, but in the larger perspective of professions in general.

Internal control mechanisms are necessary for a socially responsible profession because the knowledge that gives it power is, in considerable though not complete measure, esoteric, specialized, and available only to the trained expert. Experts from other fields, as well as the general population, do not possess the knowledge that alone makes it possible to judge and control the performance of professional peers, of fellow-experts. There is probably some exaggeration on the part of experts of the inability of the outsider to understand a reasonable account of their knowledge and its consequences. Nevertheless, there remains an inevitable knowledge gap between professional expert and "the layman" which requires that there be effective mechanisms of internal control if a profession is to be socially responsible. Standards of professional competence, performance, and ethics must rest, in considerable measure, in the hands of a community of professional peers.

But external control mechanisms are also necessary for a socially responsible profession because the consequences of its performances and power are

---

[3] See Talcott Parsons, "The Professions and Social Structure," *Social Forces*, 17 (1939): 457–467.

too important to the outsiders for them to give up all control over their fate. We now paraphrase Clemenceau's aphorism, "War is too important to be left to the generals," in many ways: medicine is too important to be left to the doctors, science is too important to be left to the scientists, and biomedical research is too important to be left to the biomedical researchers. Because the consequences of professional power are too important to be left to the professionals, outsiders ask the kind of control that comes at least from having the professionals make a reasonable effort to give a reasonable account of what they are doing. Immersed in their own special culture and activities, professionals often not only do not take the initiative in offering such accounts but are resistant to the requests of their clients that accounts be given. Moreover, in the further search for some measure of control over what is so consequential for them, the clients of professionals demand that, where internal controls are either lacking or ineffective, such controls be instituted or improved. It is this kind of search for some measure of control over biomedical research that has resulted in the mandatory requirement of peer group review and in efforts towards its improvement. For where internal controls do not exist or are not effective or cannot be made more effective, then clients will lose confidence in their professionals and will seek some kind of external control. It is our belief that one possible cause of the recent rapid rise in the number of malpractice suits against doctors in the United States is the widespread public loss of confidence in the efficacy of the internal mechanisms of control over incompetent therapeutic practice in the medical profession. Neither informal interaction processes among doctors nor the more formal processes of the ethics committees of the county medical societies are felt to be effective means of insuring social responsibility on the part of a considerable number of physicians.[4] The result is recourse to the law as an external mechanism of social control. If there ever developed a widespread feeling on the part of patients that they were being abused as subjects, there would be a similar loss of confidence in the biomedical research profession and a similar recourse to malpractice or battery suits or other forms of external control, legal or legislative. Loss of confidence in the

---

[4] For an analytical and empirical treatment of the problems of internal and external controls in the American medical profession, see Eliot Freidson, *Professional Dominance: The Social Structure of Medical Care* (New York: Atherton Press, 1970). For less sociological demands for more external control, see: Robert S. McCleery, M.D., ed., *One Life–One Physician: An Inquiry into the Medical Profession's Performance in Self-Regulation* (Washington, D.C.: Public Affairs Press, 1970); and also, The Health Policy Advisory Center, *The American Health Empire* (New York: Random House, 1970). Finally, for a study of some of the changing views on inside and outside regulation in a social science profession, see Gladys Engel Lang, "Professionalism under Attack: The Case of the Anthropologists," *Social Science Information*, 10 (1971): 117–132.

effectiveness of the internal controls of any profession is likely to lead to an increase in the external controls that a society puts on that profession. It is in the best interest of the norms and actual performance of any profession, therefore, to take the responsibility for making its system of internal controls as effective as possible. Nonetheless, even in this most favorable situation, some minimal external control will remain, for society will always insist at least on requiring professions to have effective internal controls. Though something like an "escapist" course of action was proposed for scientists twenty-five years ago by Norbert Wiener and more recently by Jacob Bronowski, no group of experts, no profession, can abdicate from its membership in and responsibility to society.

SOME SUGGESTIONS FOR POLICY CHANGE AND REFORM

Thus it is on this understanding—that an effective system of internal control best serves the normative and performance interests of the biomedical research profession, and that a mixture of internal and external controls is inevitable and best protects all the parties at interest—that we make some suggestions for policy change and reform. Though a few go beyond them in some measure, most of our suggestions are based directly on our findings and analysis. Therefore our suggestions are grouped and ordered according to the various social sources of conformity and deviance that we have examined in our earlier chapters.

The Competition Structures of Science and of Local Scientific Institutions. Because the prized goals for which scientists strive, priority of discovery in the larger scientific community and higher rank in their local scientific institutions, are scarce goods, competition is inevitable in the scientific community. This structure of competition has its functions; it conduces on the whole to better scientific performance. But it also has its dysfunctions, our findings show. Men who are relative failures in this competition or who feel they have been unfairly treated are more likely to express permissive standards and manifest permissive behavior in the use of human subjects.

The internal control mechanisms of biomedical science ought, therefore, to pay some attention to this structure of competition and its possibilities for producing some undesirable consequences. Medical training programs, informal interaction structures, and peer review processes all ought to take some cognizance both of the competition itself and of its undesirable consequences under certain conditions. But neither scientists at large nor biomedical scientists in particular like even to acknowledge the fact of competition, let alone its consequences. Instead of being seen for what it is, a realistic and inevitable aspect of competent performance, competition is seen as the product of warped personalities and peculiar circumstances. For scientists have two other important values besides priority of discovery which the acknowledgement of structured competition would seem to threaten. Those values are the *humility of the individual* as only a small part of the great process of scientific progress and the *communality of property* of all successes achieved by all individual scientists taken as a collectivity. Those two values are indeed in some measure threatened by competition and priority quarrels. But this measure can be kept in better bounds by acknowledging the fact of competition and seeking to control it, not by denying it. All scientists, the very best perhaps most of all, have to be and are competitive.[5]

So far as the harmful consequences for human subjects of scientific competition are concerned, we should also note that our data may not have included all the possible types of situations that are unfavorable in this respect. Our data show that it is more likely to be the "losers" than the "winners" who have permissive standards and practices. Yet we have impressionistic evidence from the public prints that there are certain conditions under which it is the "winner" type of scientist who is pressured by the structure of competition toward permissive standards in the use of human subjects. For example, where the struggle for priority of discovery among several leading scientists becomes highly visible to all of them, the competition often becomes keen, and occasionally even fierce, and there is considerable pressure toward permissive use of human subjects. It has been suggested in the medical and public press that just this kind of situation has occurred in the competition for priority in the heart transplant procedure and in the artificial heart program.[6] The structure of competition works in many different ways but it includes all scientists. It is clear that all the social control mechanisms for biomedical science, internal and external, will have to take competition and its undesirable consequences into account.

Socialization Structures and Processes. During the last fifty years, as the practice of medicine has become ever more pervasively scientific, the substance of medical training at all levels, from medical school through clinical internships and residencies, has ever more heavily been made up of the scientific knowledge without which modern medical practice is now impossible. Going along with this great inculcation of the scientific substance has been a large emphasis on the value of scientific research in medicine. Our data show that the medical schools have been effective in training their students into the value of research.

---

[5] For a participant account of the competition structure of science, see J. D. Watson, *The Double Helix* (New York: Atheneum, 1968). For a sociological account, see the works by Merton, Hagstrom, and Storer referred to in Chapter 4, footnote 2.

[6] See Thomas Thompson, *Hearts: Of Surgeons and Transplants. Miracles and Disasters Along the Cardiac Frontier* (New York: McCall, 1972).

But when we look at the other side of medical training, when we look for the socialization into the ethics of the use of human subjects in the research that is so highly valued, we find a different and less favorable picture. With regard to ethical training, either formal or informal, either intended or unintended, as our data show, both the medical schools and the teaching-and-research hospitals in which future researchers are trained in internships and residencies have been laggard in their obligations. Nowhere do we find any evidence of serious training or even any serious discussion of what such training ought to include.

Improvement in ethical socialization is desirable at every phase of medical training. In medical school, for example, the teachers who now instill the value of research as they talk about their own research projects ought to address themselves in proper measure to the ethical problems that occur in such research. For it is only when medical students see that their teachers are taking research ethics as a continuing and serious concern that they will themselves come to define it in the same way. In a more formal way, though we know well that the medical school curriculum is crowded and is endlessly under siege from "important" newcomers to knowledge, it is desirable that there be at least some short courses in biomedical research ethics. The teaching vehicle for such courses is now, fortunately, at hand in the form of the systematic book of cases and readings on the ethics of research compiled by Dr. Jay Katz and his colleagues.[7] Going through such a book and discussing its contents with fellow-students and an instructor would be invaluable not only for future researchers but for those many practitioners who have the ethical responsibility for the patients who become research subjects. To the extent to which such explicit training is neglected, the rights of patient-subjects will continue to be violated out of simple ignorance of the relevant norms; ignorance as a source of failure to conform to the highest standards of ethical concern ought no longer to be accepted.

Even if medical school ethical socialization were improved in these ways, like all other aspects of medical training it ought to proclaim the ideal of "continuing education." Certainly the ethical training for interns and resi-

---

[7] *Experimentation with Human Beings* (New York: Russell Sage Foundation, 1972). Further on the need for ethical education in medical schools, see the Report of the Special Committee to the Council of the Federation of American Scientists, Nov., 1967, Louis Lasagna, Roy E. Ritts, and Maurice B. Visscher, Chairman. The last sentence of this Report says: "Institutions in which human subject research is performed, especially the medical schools and the research hospitals, should make the entire subject of ethics in human experimentation a part of their regular educational programs."

For a report on some new efforts in the teaching of medical ethics in general, see *The Hastings Center Report*, 2, no. 1 (Feb., 1972) (published by the Institute of Society, Ethics, and Life Sciences, Hastings-on-Hudson, New York).

dents in teaching-and-research hospitals needs to be improved. Ethics seminars that go beyond the medical school discussions would be especially appropriate in the midst of the large amount of ongoing research that characterizes these hospitals. And finally, still under the aegis of the ideal of "continuing education," mature researchers would do well to take it as an endless task to learn about new ethical problems and new versions of old ethical problems, for that seems in fact to be the situation of scientific research using human subjects. As biomedical science progresses, some new ethical problems come up and some old ones take on new shapes. Both in science and in research ethics there get to be some more and more easy answers, but there always remains also something new to learn.

Collaboration Groups and Informal Interaction Structures. As we saw in Chapter 8, modern biomedical research is highly collaborative; in our Intensive Two-Institution Study almost 81% of the studies using human subjects involve two or more researchers. The collaboration group, then, and the other informal interaction structures that make up the immediate social environment of these researchers constitute one of the primary sites of social control. This specific finding for biomedical research only confirms a more general sociological finding that the small social groups in which human beings work, play, and carry on a great many other social activities are essential agencies for socialization and social control.

Our data also show, unfortunately, that the "climate" of these biomedical collaboration groups is more favorable to the position that we have called "value of research" than it is to the "humane therapy" position. Our data show that while such characteristics of researchers as "scientific ability" (86%) and "motivation to work hard" (45%) are highly salient to those choosing collaborators, "ethical concern for research subjects" (6%) is at the other extreme of salience. Though other data show that the "humane therapy" value in choosing collaborators may be there in latent form, since we know that some researchers tend to choose their ethical similars, still it is clear that here again we see how modern biomedical research has tended to emphasize scientific accomplishment more than ethical concern for the subjects used in scientific research. A greater preoccupation with the "ethical concern for research subjects" on the part of all collaborators would seem to be an indispensable requisite for more effective ethical practice and control among the members of biomedical research groups. Here is a definite focus for needed reform. For the immediate present, even a few highly ethically aware individuals could be of great benefit to their collaborators. In the longer run, an improved ethical socialization in medical school ought to train all future researchers in the desirability of valuing ethical concern in their research associates.

Not only the "climate" of collaboration groups but also aspects of their structure seem to be in need of improvement for more effective ethical practice. In our less systematic data, and especially in the kinds of case materials presented in Chapter 8, it became apparent that many senior bio-medical research personnel were only nominally the "principal investigators" that they were presented as being to funding agencies and other bodies. While general sponsorship by seniors of junior and less distinguished men has its positive functions in scientific research, still this sponsorship is assumed to be at least sufficient to guarantee certain acceptable standards of perform-ance. Both scientific performance and ethical performance in the case of research using human subjects should be thus guaranteed. Our cases show several instances in which senior sponsors have been so out of touch with the particular collaboration groups in which they are the nominal principal investigators that they often do not even remember that nominal connection. It is unlikely that such "members" of collaboration groups would provide even the minimal amounts of scientific and ethical supervision and partici-pation that are necessary for achieving a high standard of performance in both of these respects. It is clear that some reform in the role of principal investigators should be looked to by funding and other agencies that are concerned for scientific and ethical standards.

Peer Group Review. As we saw in Chapter 9, peer group review is the set of formally defined structures and processes that various governmental agencies and individual biomedical research organizations have stipulated as necessary for producing normatively desirable performance with regard to the use of human subjects by their grantees or individual members or con-stituent collaboration groups. We have suggested that this is the type of rele-vant social control where probably the largest changes have occurred in recent years and with probably the most favorable effects for ethical stand-ards and practices. But our data in Chapter 9 also showed that there is still serious need for improvement in the use of this valuable new social invention.

Our detailed findings and analysis in Chapter 9 spell out where such improvement should be made. There is no need to repeat Chapter 9 here; it reports a whole set of less than entirely satisfactory fulfillments, and a few decidedly unsatisfactory ones, of the already stipulated requirements of peer group review and specifies a set of conditions, not yet always stipulated by the mandating agencies, under which peer group review seems to be more rather than less efficacious. Chapter 9 provides many useful guides to policy change and reform. Perhaps it remains only to highlight one or two of the points already made and to explore somewhat more intensively a point which has been touched upon but not sufficiently explored. That is the point about the use of "outsiders" on peer review committees.

First, then, we may highlight a few needed reforms indicated in Chap-ter 9. It is clear that *all* research using human subjects should be reviewed in all institutions. Not only is such universal review required by biomedical research commitment to the highest ethical standards, but our findings seem to show that such universal review may be one of the conditions of greater efficacy for peer review. Morality and efficacy, for once, seem to coincide in the same process. Another needed reform, a connected one, is that both research institutions themselves and review-mandating organizations should study more carefully than they yet have just what constitutes "research." Granted that in an innovative field like biomedical research using human subjects the line between the "standard" and the "experimental" and between the "trivial" and the "consequential" is often hard to draw, still it would appear that not enough serious study has been given to the problem of drawing the line. In the meantime, more rather than fewer researchers can wittingly or unwittingly evade the requirement that all research be reviewed. Certainly it is desirable to be cautious, to give the patient-subject the benefit of every doubt and have rather more than less of what is tried out on him exposed to the scrutiny of peers. A closer approximation than now exists to peer group review of "all research" is much to be desired.

Now, with a view to some needed reforms in this area, we should like to explore a little more fully than we could in Chapter 9 the role of "outsiders" on peer review groups. Earlier in this chapter we tried to show why a mixture of internal and external controls is desirable in regulating the activities of a powerful profession like biomedical research. One of the appropriate sites for such a mixture of controls is the peer review committee, where not only the esoteric activities and special interests of researchers are at issue but also the special interests and moral welfare of patient-subjects. The essential role of the nonresearcher "outsider" on the committee is indicated by the following stipulation in the latest H.E.W. (which includes N.I.H.) guide to the desirable composition of such committees:

> In addition to possessing the professional competence to review specific activities, the committee should be able to determine acceptability of the proposal in terms of institutional commitments and regulations, applicable law, standards of professional conduct and practice, and community attitudes. The committee may therefore need to include persons whose primary concerns lie in these areas rather than in the conduct of research, development, and service programs of the types supported by the DHEW.[8]

But our data show that outsiders of all kinds are not common on local-institutional peer review committees. Our National Survey shows that only 10% of the responding institutions said they had members on their com-

---

[8] U.S. Department of Health, Education, and Welfare, *The Institutional Guide to DHEW Policy on Protection of Human Subjects, Dec. 1, 1971* (Washington, D.C.: U.S. Government Printing Office, 1971).

mittees from other institutions who do clinical research in the general areas in which members of these institutions themselves do research; 10% use M.D.'s from other institutions who do no clinical research in the reporting institutions' areas of specialization. As for other kinds of outsiders, 4% use lawyers who are not in their employ; 5% use behavioral scientists not in their employ; and 4% use clergymen. Only one institution has a patient sitting on its peer review committee. Altogether, only 22% of our sample of institutions have any kind of outsider, that is, nonmember of the institution, as a committee member.

We have already said that more of the specialist outsiders ought to be members of the committees, more of the researchers from other institutions who know about the specialized research projects under review but who are free of the personal and particularist connections that inevitably build up among colleagues in any given local institution and that interfere in some measure with objective judgment. Friendship has its place, but there can be too much of it on a peer review group. In the presence of a competent outsider, even friends are glad to be completely objective.

Because of the dilemma of science and therapy, some reformers have advocated that different persons play the role of clinical investigator and the role of physician with respect to every patient-subject, in order to prevent or reduce role-conflict and to protect better the rights and welfare of the patient-subject.[9] This seems to be a good way to structure the situation whenever it is possible, but unfortunately it is not always a practicable or practical possibility. As a probably more practical although perhaps less effective alternative, at least one member of every peer review committee should be a knowledgeable clinician who is not engaged in research[10] and who preferably is an outsider.

Representation of nonprofessional outsiders is also very much needed. The "community," meaning either the local community or the society as a whole, does have, as the DHEW Guide says, an important stake in what is going on. Perhaps the biomedical research profession has been slow to make nonprofessional outsiders members of its review committees because it was aware of the difficulty of finding suitable ones. It is not hard to see that it is difficult, perhaps impossible, to find one person, or even a few, who are adequately representative of the full diversity of the local community or the society. Certainly the clergyman, who seems to be the favored type of non-

---

[9] See, for example, O. E. Guttentag, "The Problems of Experimentation on Human Beings: The Physician's Point of View," *Science*, 117 (1953):204–210.

[10] M. H. Pappworth, *Human Guinea Pigs* (Boston: Beacon Press, 1968), p. 208. For another statement of proposed solutions to the dilemma of science and therapy, see Stewart E. Perry, *The Human Nature of Science* (New York: Free Press, 1966), Appendix.

professional outsider when outsiders are used at all, can probably not claim to be an adequate representative of the larger public.

The biomedical research profession has perhaps been inhospitable to nonprofessional outsiders on its review committees also because of its awareness that a certain degree and kind of informed participation was essential to effective service. In discussions where the use of nonprofessional outsiders is recommended, no specification of them is given except some vague representation of community attitudes. In an extreme view, it might sometimes seem as if the uninformed man-in-the-street was being recommended. There would not be much use in such members, and well might professional researchers think so and fear the harm a person of that kind would do to their interests and the interests of their patient-subjects.

What would seem desirable in this situation is the invention of a new social role, that of informed outsider, a role that could more effectively represent the values and interests of all who have stakes in the proceedings of the review committees, not only the patient-subjects and future patients but the research profession itself. What different kinds of knowledge and experience would be required in this new social role? First, some knowledge would be required of the nature of biomedical research, of some of its principles, methods, and substance. Second, some knowledge is needed of the laws, codes, and norms relevant to the ethical use of human subjects, and also some knowledge of the principles of effective functioning of the kind of quasi-judicial committees that the review groups in fact are. And, third, there is the need for some knowledge of the new techniques of survey research available for discovering what the values and feelings of a representative sample of the population are about biomedical research in general and any important specific new research in particular. The uninformed man-in-the-street cannot know what "the community" thinks about catheterization of the heart, or the use of levodopa in the treatment of parkinsonism, or the transplantation of vital organs, or the injection of live cancer cells into terminal cancer patients. The informed outsider would have access to the techniques and the resources that could provide such information from the community.

Where might recruits come from for such a new role? Some physicians at various stages of their career might wish to switch to this new occupation and acquire the additional training necessary for it. Or some lawyers might similarly like to switch and make this another one of the specialties into which lawyers in our society eventually go. Or some nurses might like to consider this new specialty. Or, finally, though they would need more training probably than any of the foregoing types of likely recruits, unspecialized college graduates might like to choose a career in this field.

How would the occupants of this new social role be trained? A special professional school or a training program for this kind of role could be set up, a school in which the training communicated the several kinds of knowledge that we have indicated are necessary and in which various opportunities for "case instruction" and apprenticeship experience were available. Such a school or program might be set up in close association with the law and medical schools of a given university. In addition, on-the-job training and experience, which is always so important for effective professional performance, would be part of the necessary socialization of the informed outsider who would be a valuable member of the peer review process.

The occupants of this new social role would not, of course, function just as individual professionals. They would, like other professionals, join in an association to improve training, maintain performance standards, and provide collective information and resources necessary for the effective performance of the new role. For example, such an association might sponsor the research on public values and feelings about some new kind of biomedical research on human subjects that its individual members needed to feed into the review process in their own local institutions.

In sum, through the medium of such a new social role, the role of professionalized and informed outsider, the community could become the active and effective moral peers in the peer review process of the biomedical researchers who now are its dominant members. If biomedical research is to have the necessary social support from all those whose values and interests are at stake, then there must be a true moral community to provide this support. In this enterprise of biomedical research, we are all either scientific peers or moral peers or both. If the community and society come to feel that they do not have effective moral participation in this enterprise, they will turn against it in some degree. The introduction of the role of informed outsider might forestall the possibility of a hostile public reaction against biomedical research. And while this new role will have costs, the costs are well worth paying both to realize our values and to forestall this possibility.

The Medical Schools. In this list of suggestions for policy change and reform we come now, finally and briefly, to the medical schools. In Chapter 10 we indicated why the medical school, like all types of professional schools, must have a central place in maintaining not only the standards of technical performance of its profession but also its values and standards of ethical performance. We have also seen that medical schools, at least in the recent past, have done better at technical training and at advancing the values and substance of scientific research than they have done in maintaining appropriate concern and performance with regard to the ethical use of human subjects in research. We suggest that it is time for a change of policy on the part of the medical schools. While preserving their proud achievements in technical training and in research, they should be paying more attention to the several different aspects of satisfactory ethical performance with regard to human subjects: they should be training their students better in his area, they should look to better training also of the interns and residents in the hospitals they supervise, they should pay more attention to peer review group performance, and they should lead the way in the study and improvement of all these important social control processes. Without this essential change of policy on the part of the medical schools, we are likely to have further demands for external controls on biomedical research and more hostility to it, at the expense of both scientific and public interests and values.

The Continuing Quest. The quest for more ethical behavior in any area of human action is inevitably a difficult and continuing one. It is a quest, certainly, that proceeds better with as much reliable information as possible about whatever field is in question. Looking back over the recent past, we feel that the continuing quest for more ethical behavior in the use of human subjects in biomedical research is well begun. We hope we have shown what sociology can contribute to this quest and that others will now join us in providing better information and analysis in this field.

APPENDIX I
NATIONAL SURVEY QUESTIONNAIRE

<u>Important</u>: Please check here if you wish to receive a summary of our research (probably in 1970): ( )

<u>CHARACTERISTICS OF YOUR INSTITUTION</u>

1. Is your institution considered to be <u>primarily</u>: (Check only <u>one</u>)

      ( ) a.   Public
      ( ) b.   Voluntary, non-profit
      ( ) c.   Private, profit
      ( ) d.   Other (please specify) _____

    1A.   <u>IF YOU CHECKED "a" ABOVE</u>, is your institution:

        ( ) 1.   A city or municipal institution
        ( ) 2.   A county institution
        ( ) 3.   A state institution
        ( ) 4.   A federal institution
        ( ) 5.   Other (please specify) _____

2. Which of the following most accurately describes your institution? (Check only <u>one</u>)

      ( ) a.   Non-teaching general hospital
      ( ) b.   Teaching hospital - no medical school
      ( ) c.   Teaching hospital - medical school
      ( ) d.   Psychiatric or mental hospital
      ( ) e.   Research institute with patients in residence
      ( ) f.   Out-patient clinic
      ( ) g.   Other (please specify) _____

    2A.   <u>IF YOUR INSTITUTION HAS PATIENTS IN RESIDENCE OR IS AN OUT-PATIENT CLINIC</u>, <u>roughly</u>, what percentage of your total patient population is:

      2A.1.   Upper class   ____%
               Upper-middle class   ____%
               Lower-middle class   ____%
               Lower class   ____%

                           (100%)

      2A.2.   Children ____%

      2A.3.   Older people beyond 60 ____%

      2A.4.   Psychiatric or mental patients ____%

      2A.5.   Terminal patients ____%

3. Is your institution effectively (as opposed to nominally) affiliated with a religious group? (Check only <u>one</u>)

    ( ) a. Yes
    ( ) b. No

    3A. <u>IF YES</u>, please specify the religious group: _____
    _____

CHARACTERISTICS OF CLINICAL RESEARCHERS AND THEIR WORK

4. We will be asking about clinical research and clinical researchers through much of this questionnaire. Is the following definition of clinical research personally acceptable to you without addition or deletion?

    <u>Clinical Research or Investigation</u>: Anything done to a person which is as yet not established, by clinical experience or scientific research, as being for his direct therapeutic benefit or as contributing to the diagnosis of his disease. (What is done may eventually, of course, be for the person's own direct or indirect therapeutic benefit and/or for the eventual therapeutic benefit of the population at large.) Investigations which involve the analysis of human substances collected as a by-product of established diagnostic or other procedures should be included here as clinical research.

    ( ) a. Yes
    ( ) b. No

    4A. <u>IF NO</u>, how would you qualify or change the above definition? (Please specify) _____
    _____
    _____
    _____

5. With which of the following statements do you most closely agree? (Check only <u>one</u>)

    ( ) a. This institution strongly encourages those who are qualified to engage in clinical research to do so.
    ( ) b. This institution moderately encourages those who are qualified to engage in clinical research to do so.
    ( ) c. This institution only slightly encourages those who are qualified to engage in clinical research to do so.
    ( ) d. This institution does not encourage those who are qualified to engage in clinical research to do so.

6. It is recognized that most research breaks new ground. But, certain kinds of research problems are often referred to as being at the "scientific frontier." Has there been any <u>clinical</u> research done in your institution <u>within the past three years</u> which you feel is of this highly original "frontier" type?

      ( ) a. Yes
      ( ) b. No

6A. <u>IF YES</u>, briefly specify one such study and give the reference to the publication if you can: _____
_____
_____
_____

7. What proportion of the <u>clinical</u> researchers in your institution work alone (aided only by technicians)? (Check only <u>one</u>)

      ( ) a. All or almost all
      ( ) b. About three-fourths
      ( ) c. About half
      ( ) d. About one-fourth
      ( ) e. None or almost none

8. If you were to add up the number of papers reporting <u>clinical</u> investigations published in 1968 by the clinical researchers in your institution to get a total for the institution as a whole, <u>according to your best estimate</u> what would the number be?

        _____ papers

8A. When it comes to the volume of clinical research done, according to your own standards, would you say that the clinical researchers in your institution are:

      ( ) 1. Highly productive
      ( ) 2. Moderately productive
      ( ) 3. Fairly productive
      ( ) 4. Relatively unproductive

8B. When it comes to their degree of concern about being productive, would you say that the clinical researchers in your institution are:

      ( ) 1. Very concerned about their productivity
      ( ) 2. Moderately concerned about their productivity
      ( ) 3. Fairly concerned about their productivity
      ( ) 4. Relatively unconcerned about their productivity

9. What sort of training do the principal <u>clinical</u> investigators and their main colleagues in your institution have? (Check only <u>one</u>)

( ) a. All M.D.'s
( ) b. Predominantly M.D.'s, some Ph.D.'s
( ) c. An almost equal number of M.D.'s and Ph.D.'s
( ) d. Predominantly Ph.D.'s, some M.D.'s
( ) e. All Ph.D.'s
( ) f. Other (please specify) _____

10. <u>Roughly,</u> what percentage of the clinical investigations done in your institution fall into each of the following categories of risk for the subjects (it is assumed that the risk is generally balanced or exceeded by the possible immediate or eventual benefits to the subjects or to the population at large):

a. A large amount of risk for the subjects ___%
b. A moderate amount of risk for the subjects ___%
c. Some risk for the subjects ___%
d. Very little or no risk for the subjects ___%

(100%)

10A. <u>IF ANY PROPORTION FALLS INTO "a" OR "b" ABOVE,</u> could you indicate what it was about one of these investigations that you feel made it risky for the subjects: _____
_____
_____

11. To what extent would you agree or disagree with the following statement?

"In your institution clinical investigators generally highly value the rights and welfare of the human subjects involved in their research."

( ) a. Very strongly agree
( ) b. Strongly agree
( ) c. Moderately agree
( ) d. Slightly agree
( ) e. Neither disagree nor agree
( ) f. Moderately disagree
( ) g. Strongly disagree

12. Which of the following categories of people are ever utilized <u>in experimental or in control</u> groups by clinical researchers in your institution? Please <u>do not include</u> persons from whom materials such as blood or urine are taken for experiment-related analysis as a by-product of regular diagnostic or other procedures. (Check <u>all</u> categories that apply)

( ) a. Patients for whom it is hoped the investigation will have <u>immediate</u> therapeutic benefits
( ) b. Patients for whom the investigation may have <u>eventual</u> therapeutic benefits, but who are primarily subjects of scientific research
( ) c. Patients whose condition is unrelated to the investigation
( ) d. The researcher himself, or other researchers
( ) e. Medical students
( ) f. Laboratory personnel or other employees of the institution
( ) g. Prisoners
( ) h. Other (please specify) _____

_____

13. Which category of subjects, already checked in question 12, is to the best of your knowledge the <u>one most often utilized</u> by the clinical researchers in your institution? Place in the following space the <u>letter</u> of the appropriate category: _____

14. In question 2A we asked you about the demographic characteristics of your patient population, if any. Now we wish to ask the same question about your clinical research subjects. <u>Roughly</u>, what percentage of the clinical research subjects in your institution are:

14A. Upper class   ____%
      Upper-middle class   ____%
      Lower-middle class   ____%
      Lower class   ____%

                          (100%)

14B. Children ____%

14C. Older people beyond 60 ____%

14D. Psychiatric or mental patients ____%

14E. Terminal patients ____%

15. To what degree would you say the rights and welfare of human subjects are safeguarded in clinical research conducted by investigators in your institution? (Check only <u>one</u>)

    ( ) a. To an outstanding degree
    ( ) b. To an extremely high degree
    ( ) c. To a very high degree
    ( ) d. To a high degree
    ( ) e. To a more than adequate degree
    ( ) f. To an adequate degree
    ( ) g. To a minimal degree

ORGANIZATION AND PROCEDURES OF THE INSTITUTIONAL REVIEW COMMITTEE

16. What was the month and year in which your institution gave formal assurance to the National Institutes of Health that an institutional review procedure complying with their guidelines for research using human subjects was in operation in your institution? Month _____ Year _____

17. In your institution, was there a review procedure which scrutinized the ethical aspects of proposed clinical research before the National Institutes of Health required that one be put into effect?

    ( ) a. Yes
    ( ) b. No

17A. IF YES TO 17, did the previous review procedure which scrutinized the ethical aspects of proposed clinical research meet the requirements of the National Institutes of Health to the degree that no changes in the procedure were required?

    ( ) 1. Yes, no revisions were required by NIH or made by this institution.
    ( ) 2. Yes, no revisions were required by NIH, but this institution took the opportunity to make some changes.
    ( ) 3. No, one or more minor changes were required by NIH.
    ( ) 4. No, one or more major changes were required by NIH.

17B. IF YES TO 17, was the pre-NIH review procedure instituted as a response to some ethical crisis in your own institution or elsewhere? (Some institutions, for example, set up review procedures on their own after the "live cancer cell injection" incident.)

    ( ) 1. Yes
    ( ) 2. No

17B.1. <u>IF YES TO 17B</u>, please specify the nature of the ethical crisis: _____

_____
_____
_____

<u>NOTE</u>: We will be referring often from here on to a committee in your organization which we will call the "institutional review committee." By this we mean that committee of associates or colleagues, required by the National Institutes of Health as a condition for obtaining their grants, which reviews the ethical aspects of clinical research using human subjects in your institution. <u>IF YOUR INSTITUTION HAS MORE THAN ONE COMMITTEE, PLEASE ANSWER THE FOLLOWING QUESTIONS WITH RESPECT TO THE ONE TO WHICH YOU REFERRED IN YOUR ASSURANCE TO NIH</u>.

18. How many members (including the chairman) does your institutional review committee have? _____ members

19. Write in the <u>number</u> of members of the institutional review committee who fall into <u>each</u> of the following categories:

      a. Members of your institution who actually engage in clinical investigation themselves _____
      b. Members of your institution who <u>do not</u> engage in clinical investigation themselves:

            1. Administrators
            2. Lawyers employed by your institution _____
            3. Members of the Board of Trustees _____
            4. Nurses _____
            5. Other (please specify) _____ _____

            _____

      c. Non-members of your institution who do clinical research in the general areas of specialization in which the members of your organization also do research _____
      d. Non-members of your institution who do <u>no</u> clinical research in your institution's general areas of specialization but who are members of the medical profession _____
      e. Non-members of your institution who are not members of the medical profession:

            1. Lawyers
            2. Social Scientists _____
            3. Clergymen _____
            4. Patients _____
            5. Other (please specify) _____ _____

            _____

20. Does your institution have one or more pathologists on the staff?

        ( ) a. Yes
        ( ) b. No

  20A. IF YES, is a pathologist a member of the institutional review committee?

        ( ) 1. Yes
        ( ) 2. No

21. From what level of the formal institutional hierarchy (including the clinical, administrative, and/or academic) do most of the members of the institutional review committee come? (Check the one which best applies)

        ( ) a. Highest level
        ( ) b. Intermediate level
        ( ) c. Lower level

22. Are there any members of your institution who spend "full time" on activities of the institutional review committee?

        ( ) a. Yes
        ( ) b. No

  22A. IF YES, check all that apply:

        ( ) 1. Full time chairman or executive secretary
        ( ) 2. Full time clerical secretary
        ( ) 3. Other (please specify) _____

    22A.1. IF THERE IS A FULL TIME CHAIRMAN OR EXECUTIVE SECRETARY, what is his occupational training and experience? (For example, you might say: internal medicine with research background; or, legal with experience in practice and administration; etc.): _____

23. Is the institutional review committee itself specialized in any way into subcommittees, departmental committees, or·an executive committee; or, are there other review committees dealing with the ethical aspects of clinical research in your institution? (Check all that apply)

    ( ) a. Subcommittees
    ( ) b. Departmental committees
    ( ) c. Executive committee
    ( ) d. Other review committees dealing with the ethical aspects of clinical research (i.e., there are committees at affiliated institutions, or at a higher or lower level in your institution)
    ( ) e. Not specialized
    ( ) f. Other (please specify) _____

  23A. IF YOU CHECKED "a", please specify the types of subcommittees: _____
_____
_____

  23B. IF YOU CHECKED "d", please specify the types: _____
_____

24. In addition to the review committee, are there any other institutional controls, formal or informal, over the ethical aspects of clinical research in your institution? (For example: the department chairman may have to review proposals first; or, the Board of Trustees may have to approve proposals.)

    ( ) a. Yes
    ( ) b. No

  24A. IF YES, could you briefly describe these additional controls: _____
_____
_____

25. Does the institutional review committee also: (Check all that apply)

    ( ) a. Allocate local research funds to clinical investigators in your institution
    ( ) b. Evaluate and review the scientific merit of proposed clinical research
    ( ) c. Neither of the above

26. How effective, would you say, is the operation of your institutional review committee in helping to protect the rights and welfare of the human subjects of clinical research in your institution? (Check only <u>one</u>)

    ( ) a. Very effective
    ( ) b. Effective to a degree
    ( ) c. Ineffective because it has little power
    ( ) d. Much of the clinical research that is actually done does not get submitted to the committee for review
    ( ) e. Other (please specify _____

27. What research is reviewed by the institutional review committee? (Check only <u>one</u>)

    ( ) a. All clinical research
    ( ) b. Only clinical research which involves a formal proposal for funds, either for funds from your institution's research budget or for funds from an external institution or agency
    ( ) c. Only formal proposals to do clinical research which involve requests for money from the Public Health Service
    ( ) d. Other (please specify) _____

28. What kind of consent does your institutional review committee require each clinical investigator to obtain from his potential subject-volunteers? (Check only <u>one</u>)

    ( ) a. Oral
    ( ) b. Written
    ( ) c. Other (please specify) _____

29. In the case of proposals for funds for clinical research from the Public Health Service, are the proposals reviewed prior to submitting the application to PHS, prior to funding but after application, or not until after the applications have been approved for funding by PHS? (Check <u>all</u> that apply)

    ( ) a. Prior to application
    ( ) b. Prior to funding but after application
    ( ) c. Subsequent to funding

30. Which of the following procedures apply to your institutional review committee? (Check <u>all</u> that apply)

    ( ) a. Committee meets as a body after pre-review of clinical research proposals by the members, by a sub-group of the members, or by an individual member. (<u>IF CHECKED, GO TO 30A</u>)
    ( ) b. Committee meets as a body with no pre-review of clinical research proposals by any of the members. (<u>IF CHECKED, GO TO 30A</u>)
    ( ) c. Other (please <u>specify</u> and then <u>GO TO 30B</u>) ____

30A.   IF THE INSTITUTIONAL REVIEW COMMITTEE MEETS AS A BODY:

    30A.1. How often does it generally meet? _____ time(s) per year

    30A.2. Roughly how many clinical research proposals are generally acted upon at a committee meeting? _____ proposals per meeting

30B.   IF THE INSTITUTIONAL REVIEW COMMITTEE DOES NOT MEET AS A BODY, approximately how many clinical research proposals does it review, say, in a three month period? _____ proposals per three month period

31. Is there a continuing review of the clinical investigations which the institutional review committee has approved? (Check only one)

    ( ) a. Yes, a continuing formal review by the committee (IF CHECKED, GO TO 31A)
    ( ) b. Yes, continuing informal review by the committee (IF CHECKED, GO TO 31B)
    ( ) c. No continuing review by the committee
    ( ) d. Other (please specify) _____
    _____

31A. IF CONTINUING FORMAL REVIEW, please specify the nature of the review and how frequently each project is reviewed: _____
_____

31B. IF CONTINUING INFORMAL REVIEW, please specify the nature of the review and how frequently each project is reviewed: _____
_____

32. What proportion of the membership of the institutional review committee is required for approval of proposed clinical research? (Check only one)

    ( ) a. Unanimity among those voting
    ( ) b. Two-thirds majority of those voting
    ( ) c. Simple majority of those voting
    ( ) d. Some other proportion (please specify) _____
    ( ) e. No specific proportion stipulated by our procedure

32A. Do you agree of disagree with the following:

"In practice, when our institutional review committee approves a clinical research proposal, it is almost always by a unanimous decision. If even one member has serious questions about the ethical aspects of such a proposal, we would probably either table the discussion, require revisions to satisfy the dissenting member, or even reject the proposal."

( ) 1. Agree
( ) 2. Disagree
( ) 3. Can't say

33. Some institutions have changed their review procedures concerning the ethical aspects of proposed clinical research in various ways subsequent to submitting their initial assurance to NIH. Is the procedure you have just been describing identical to the one that existed when your institution submitted its assurance to NIH; or, have there been changes in the procedure since then?

( ) a. The review procedure is the same as the one which existed when our institution submitted its assurance.
( ) b. There have been changes in the review procedure since our institution submitted its assurance.

33A. IF YOU CHECKED "b" ABOVE, PLEASE ANSWER THE FOLLOWING QUESTION: When did the latest modification in your institution's review procedure take place? Month _____ _____ Year _____

34. Are the review procedures concerning the ethical aspects of proposed clinical research in your institution in writing?

( ) a. Yes
( ) b. No

THE COMMITTEE'S EXPERIENCE SO FAR

35. With respect to the ethical aspects of the proposed
clinical research which has come before your institutional
review committee, which of the following apply? (Check <u>all</u>
that apply)

      ( ) a. The committee <u>has not</u> required any revisions
            of proposed clinical research for ethical
            reasons.

      ( ) b. The committee <u>has</u> required researchers to re-
            vise their proposed clinical research for
            ethical reasons in one or more cases, but
            after revision these <u>were all approved</u>.

      ( ) c. The committee <u>has</u> required researchers to re-
            vise their proposed clinical research for
            ethical reasons in one or more cases, but
            after revision <u>one or more of these were re-
            jected</u>.

      ( ) d. There have been one or more rejections of pro-
            posed clinical research by the committee for
            ethical reasons.

      ( ) e. There have been one or more instances where
            an investigator withdrew his proposal when he
            sensed that revision or rejection for ethical
            reasons was likely.

   35A. <u>IF YOU CHECKED "b" or "c" IN QUESTION 35</u>:

      35A.1. According to your best estimate, what percent-
            age of clinical research proposals coming be-
            fore your committee require revision for eth-
            ical reasons: _____ %

      35A.2. Can you very briefly give an example of such a
            proposed clinical investigation which required
            revision for ethical reasons and the specific
            reasons the revision was required? <u>Example</u>:

            _____
            _____

   35B. <u>IF YOU CHECKED "c" or "d" IN QUESTION 35</u>:

      35B.1. According to your best estimate, what percent-
            age of clinical research proposals coming before
            your committee have been rejected for ethical
            reasons: _____ %

      35B.2. Can you very briefly give an example of a pro-
            posed clinical investigation which the commit-
            tee has rejected for ethical reasons and the
            specific reasons approval was withheld?
            <u>Example</u>: _____

            _____
            _____

35C. IF YOU CHECKED "e" IN QUESTION 35:

    35C.1. According to your best estimate, what percentage of clinical research proposals coming before your committee were withdrawn by the investigator when he sensed that revision or rejection for ethical reasons was likely: _____%

36. If your committee recommends revision or rejection for a clinical research proposal on ethical grounds, is there any _formal_ way that the investigator can appeal the decision of the committee?

    ( ) a. Yes
    ( ) b. No

36A. IF YES, please specify the official person(s) or group to whom he can appeal: _____

37. Does the institutional review committee find that proposed clinical research, rejected or needing modification on ethical grounds, generally also lacks merit on purely scientific grounds? (Check _all_ that apply)

    ( ) a. Yes, generally also lacks merit on substantive scientific grounds.
    ( ) b. Yes, generally also lacks merit on methodological grounds.
    ( ) c. No, generally has merit on substantive scientific grounds.
    ( ) d. No, generally has merit on methodological grounds.
    ( ) e. There seems to be no relation between scientific merit and ethical questions generally.
    ( ) f. Other (please specify) _____

38. Generally speaking, would you say that the work of the institutional review committee _with respect to its review of the ethical aspects of clinical research_ has been well received by the clinical researchers in your institution? Please _do not_ include as opposition such things as the common complaint about increased paperwork.

    ( ) a. Very well received
    ( ) b. Fairly well received, no opposition
    ( ) c. Some opposition to the work of the committee
    ( ) d. Much opposition to the work of the committee
    ( ) e. Other (please specify) _____

39. According to your best estimate, how much consensus is there among the members of the institutional review committee on the general ethical issues associated with clinical research? (Check only <u>one</u>)

    ( ) a. The members of the committee have almost identical positions on the general ethical issues associated with clinical research.

    ( ) b. There are some very minor differences in position among the members.

    ( ) c. There are some major differences in position among the members.

40. Has your institutional review committee ever consulted with the same committee in another institution for any purpose (e.g., concerning procedural matters when the committee was first being set up, or some substantive issue in deciding a case)?

    ( ) a. Yes
    ( ) b. No

  40A. <u>IF YES</u>, briefly describe the purpose of one such consultation: _____

_____

SOME PROPOSED CLINICAL INVESTIGATIONS FOR REVIEW

The following is a set of hypothetical research proposals. <u>Please assume that these proposed clinical investigations have never been conducted before</u> - that is, they would not be replications of research already done (even if you know that any of them actually have been done before). With respect to each, we would like to know: (1) in the hypothetical case that you constituted an institutional review "committee of one," what decision you would make after reviewing the proposal; (2) what decision, according to your best estimate, the existing institutional review committee at your institution would make; (3) what opinion you feel the majority of the clinical researchers in your institution would have concerning the proposal, acting in their role as researcher rather than as a "committee of one."

41.   Researcher A is associated with a university-affiliated
medical school. He proposes by the following means to inves-
tigate the important question of the relation between the use
of hallucinogenic drugs and chromosome break among the under-
graduates at the university. Students commonly visit the
student health center for diagnosis and treatment of their
various health problems. The researcher proposes to have a
urine sample and blood test taken for experiment-related
analysis from every student who comes to the health center.
The blood test and urine sample are not a routine part of
students' visits to the health center. The volume of fluid
involved in each case is small. You know that the researcher
is highly competent, and the research design is of high quality. You believe also that the chances of an important discovery are high.

   41A. Hypothetically assuming that you constitute an institutional review "committee of one," and that the proposed research has never been done before, would you:

          ( ) 1. Approve the proposal as it stands?
          ( ) 2. Require some revisions in the proposal
                  before you would approve it?
          ( ) 3. Reject the proposal?

   41A.1. IF YOU CHECKED "2" IN 41A, what revisions or
changes would you require in the proposal before you
would approve it? _____

_____
_____
_____
_____
_____

   41A.2. IF YOU CHECKED "3" IN 41A, why would you reject
the proposal? _____

_____
_____
_____
_____
_____

41B. What do you think the existing institutional review
committee in your institution would do and their reason(s)
for doing it? _____

_____
_____
_____

41C. What opinion do you think the majority of the researchers in your institution would hold concerning the
above proposal, acting in their role as researcher rather
than as a "committee of one"? _____

_____
_____
_____

42. A congenital defect involving a hole in the wall separating the ventricles of the heart is sometimes found in children. Surgery is generally immediately called for in those cases where it is large. In cases where the hole is small, surgery is not generally required. In children in whom the hole is of an intermediate size, medical opinion differs as to the advisability of early surgery. Assuming for the purposes of this question that open heart surgery for such intermediate cases involves a risk of mortality of about 3%, and that the operation has proved successful in about 95% of the survivors, the investigator wishes to determine the presently unknown long-term risks of postponing surgery until, if ever, it becomes positively indicated.

The researcher would randomly select an experimental and a control group from a population of children with the intermediate congenital heart defect who are otherwise healthy. He would operate immediately on the experimental group and postpone surgery for the controls until, if ever, it became positively indicated. For each group he would then construct what are, essentially, life tables, by means of which one could compare not only the mortality rates but also the degree to which the children are able to function normally.

The investigator is known to be highly competent, and he plans to obtain consent to perform surgery from the parents of those children in the experimental group. He will obtain parental consent to perform surgery on any controls if there comes to be a positive indication that surgery is required at any time during the period of the investigation. He does not intend, however, to inform either group of parents that their children will be taking part in a clinical investigation.

42A. Hypothetically assuming that you constitute an institutional review "committee of one," and that the proposed research has never been done before, would you:

( ) 1. Approve the proposal as it stands?
( ) 2. Require some revisions in the proposal before you would approve it?
( ) 3. Reject the proposal?

42A.1. IF YOU CHECKED "2" IN 42A, what revisions or
changes would you require in the proposal before you
would approve it? _____
_____
_____
_____
_____
_____

42A.2. IF YOU CHECKED "3" IN 42A, why would you reject the proposal? _____
_____
_____
_____
_____

42B. What do you think the existing institutional review
committee in your institution would do and their reason(s)
for doing it? _____
_____
_____
_____

42C. What opinion do you think the majority of the researchers in your institution would hold concerning the
above proposal, acting in their role as researcher rather
than as a "committee of one"? _____
_____
_____
_____

43. A researcher in a psychiatric hospital has been asked to
test a new drug (IND Phase 2) intended for the relief of the
symptoms of severe depression. In a published uncontrolled
clinical trial involving 60 patient-subjects, 54 of the patient-subjects showed a marked improvement, 5 patient-subjects
showed little or no change, and one patient-subject appeared
to become worse. In addition, however, the new drug produced
a mild pruritic rash plus severe diarrhea in 12 of the patient-
subjects. The rash appeared shortly after administration of
the drug and disappeared spontaneously 4-6 hours later. The
diarrhea produced a loose, watery stool, appeared some 6-8
hours after the drug was administered, and lasted for approximately 6 hours. In addition, laboratory tests indicated that
there were temporary and mild changes in liver function in 2
patient-subjects with no evidence of permanent damage. There
was no evidence of bone marrow depression or other toxic effects.

The best of the approved competing drugs produces much
milder side-effects in less than 3% of the cases in which it
is used, and it has proved to be effective in alleviating the
symptoms of severe depression about 60% of the time. The researcher plans to administer the new drug to an experimental
group of severely depressed in-patients, some of whom have
suicidal tendencies, and to administer a placebo to the same
type of patient as a control group. He will attempt to determine the efficacy and safety of the new drug. The researcher,
whom you know to be highly competent, plans to obtain the
written consent of both the experimental and control patient-
subjects (if possible) or their legal guardians after explaining the nature and purposes of the investigation. He
plans to inform them, too, of the possibility of the above-
stated side-effects, and that double blind procedures will
be used.

43A. Hypothetically assuming that you constitute an institutional review "committee of one," would you:

( ) 1. Approve the proposal as it stands?
( ) 2. Require some revisions in the proposal
before you would approve it?
( ) 3. Reject the proposal?

43A.1. <u>IF YOU CHECKED "2" IN 43A</u>, what revisions or changes would you require in the proposal before you would approve it? _____

_____

_____

_____

_____

_____

43A.2. <u>IF YOU CHECKED "3" IN 43A</u>, why would you re-ject the proposal? _____

_____

_____

_____

_____

43B. What do you think the <u>existing institutional review committee</u> in your institution would do and their reason(s) for doing it? _____

_____

_____

_____

43C. What opinion do you think the <u>majority of the researchers</u> in your institution would hold concerning the above proposal, acting in their role as researcher rather than as a "committee of one"? _____

_____

_____

_____

44. It has been shown that the thymus has an important bearing on the development and maintenance of immunity. For this reason the researcher proposes an investigation to determine the effect of thymus removal on the survival of tissue transplants, a very timely and important problem. In a sample of children and adolescents admitted for surgery to correct congenital heart lesions, he would randomly select an experimental group for thymectomy. Though the thymectomy will prolong the heart surgery by a few minutes, there is otherwise extrememly little additional surgical risk from this procedure. At the conclusion of each heart operation, a full-thickness skin graft, approximately one cm. in diameter and obtained from an unrelated adult donor, would be sutured in place on the chest wall of both the experimental and control groups. He would then compare the survival of the skin grafts in each of the groups. It has been shown in a number of investigations on neonatal rats and other animals that those whose thymus had been removed were much less likely to reject skin grafts. The possible long-term immunological problems that might result are as yet not completely known, but a number of studies in animals indicate significant immunological deficiencies after thymectomy. Studies done in humans with myasthenia gravis, some of whom had undergone thymectomy, have not definitively demonstrated that the immunological abnormalities discovered in these patients were the result of thymectomies. To quote one authority: "There were no immunologic abnormalities that could be attributed to the effect of thymectomy per se."

The research will result in no therapeutic benefits for the patients involved. The researcher plans to obtain the consent of his potential patient-volunteers and/or their parents after explaining the procedures involved in the investigation as well as the possible short-term surgical and long-term immunological hazards for the subjects.

44A. Hypothetically assuming that you constitute an institutional review "committee of one," and that the proposed research has never been done before, please check the <u>lowest</u> probability that <u>you</u> would consider acceptable for <u>your</u> approval of the proposed investigation. (Check only <u>one</u>)

( ) 1. If the chances are 1 in 10 that the proposed investigation will establish that thymectomy considerably increases the probability of tissue transplant survival in children and adolescents.

( ) 2. If the chances are 3 in 10 that the proposed investigation will establish that thymectomy considerably increases the probability of tissue transplant survival in children and adolescents.

( ) 3. If the chances are 5 in 10 that the proposed investigation will establish that thymectomy considerably increases the probability of tissue transplant survival in children and adolescents.

( ) 4. If the chances are 7 in 10 that the proposed investigation will establish that thymectomy considerably increases the probability of tissue transplant survival in children and adolescents.

( ) 5. If the chances are 9 in 10 that the proposed investigation will establish that thymectomy considerably increases the probability of tissue transplant survival in children and adolescents.

( ) 6. Place a check here if you feel that, as the proposal stands, the researcher should not attempt the investigation no matter what the probability that the proposed investigation will establish that thymectomy considerably increases the chances of transplant survival in children and adolescents. (<u>IF YOU CHECKED HERE</u>, please explain): _____

_____

_____

_____

_____

44B. Which of the above responses comes closest to what you feel the existing institutional review committee in your institution would make? _____ (Please write in the number of the response.)

44C. Which of the above responses comes closest to what you feel the majority of the researchers in your institution would make, acting in their role as researcher rather than as a "committee of one"? _____ (Please write in the number of the response.)

IF YOU WOULD LIKE TO MAKE ANY COMMENTS ON ANY PART OF QUESTION 44, please use the following space: _____
_____
_____

45. A researcher plans to study bone metabolism in children suffering from a serious bone disease. He intends to determine the degree of appropriation of calcium into the bone by using radioactive calcium. In order to make an adequate comparison, he intends to use some healthy children as controls, and he plans to obtain the consent of the parents of both groups of children after explaining to them the nature and purposes of the investigation and the short and long-term risks to their children. Evidence from animals and earlier studies in humans indicates that the size of the radioactive dose to be administered here would only very slightly (say, by 5-10 chances in a million) increase the probability of the subjects involved contracting leukemia or experiencing other problems in the long run. While there is no definitive data as yet on the incidence of leukemia in children, a number of doctors and statistical sources indicate that the rate is about 250/million in persons under 18 years of age. Assume for the purpose of this question that the incidence of the bone disease being discussed is about the same as that for leukemia in children under 18 years of age. The investigation, if successful, would add greatly to medical knowledge regarding this particular bone disease, but the administration of the radioactive calcium would not be of immediate therapeutic benefit for either group of children. The results of the investigation may, however, eventually benefit the group of children suffering from the bone disease. Please assume for the purposes of this question that there is no other method that would produce the data the researcher desires. The researcher is known to be highly competent in this area.

45A. Hypothetically assuming that you constitute an institutional review "committee of one," and that the proposed investigation has **never** been done before, please check the <u>lowest</u> probability that <u>you</u> would consider acceptable for <u>your</u> approval of the proposed investigation. (Check only <u>one</u>)

( ) 1. If the chances are 1 in 10 that the investigation will lead to an important medical discovery.

( ) 2. If the chances are 3 in 10 that the investigation will lead to an important medical discovery.

( ) 3. If the chances are 5 in 10 that the investigation will lead to an important medical discovery.

( ) 4. If the chances are 7 in 10 that the investigation will lead to an important medical discovery.

( ) 5. If the chances are 9 in 10 that the investigation will lead to an important medical discovery.

( ) 6. Place a check here if you feel that, as the proposal stands, the researcher should not attempt the investigation, no matter what the probability that an important medical discovery will result. (<u>IF YOU CHECKED HERE</u>, please explain): _____

_____
_____
_____

45B. Which of the above responses comes closest to what you feel the <u>existing institutional review committee</u> in your institution would make? _____ (Please write in the number of the response.)

45C. Which of the above responses comes closest to what you feel the <u>majority of the researchers</u> in your institution would make, acting in their role as researcher rather than as a "committee of one"? _____ (Please write in the number of the response.)

IF YOU WOULD LIKE TO MAKE ANY COMMENTS ON ANY PART OF <u>QUESTION 45</u>, please use the following space: _____

_____
_____
_____

46. A researcher proposes to study pulmonary function in adults under anesthesia for routine hernia repair. In order to complete the necessary measurements for the investigation, patients would have to remain under the anesthesia for an additional half hour. The researcher plans to obtain the consent of the potential patient-volunteers after explaining to them the nature and purposes of the investigation as well as the possible risks involved. The completion of the investigation at this particular time would result in an important increase in medical knowledge of the effects of anesthesia on pulmonary function. As a result of the additional time under anesthesia, the probability of post-operative complications such as atelectasis (collapse of some pulmonary tissue) and pneumonia might increase.

46A. Hypothetically assuming that you constitute an institutional review "committee of one," and that the proposed research has never been done before, please check the <u>highest</u> probability that <u>you</u> would consider acceptable for <u>your</u> approval of the proposed investigation.

( ) 1. If there is a greater than 15% but less than 35% chance that an increase in these post-operative complications would result.

( ) 2. If there is a 15% chance that an increase in these post-operative complications would result.

( ) 3. If there is a 10% chance than an increase in these post-operative complications would result.

( ) 4. If there is a 5% chance that an increase in these post-operative complications would result.

( ) 5. If there is virtually no chance that an increase in these post-operative complications would result.

( ) 6. Place a check here if you feel that, as the proposal stands, the researcher should not attempt the investigation, no matter what the probability that an increase in these post-operative complications would result. (<u>IF YOU CHECKED HERE</u>, please explain): _____

_____
_____
_____

46B. Which of the above responses comes closest to what you feel the existing institutional review committee in your institution would make? _____ (Please write in the number of the response.)

46C. Which of the above responses comes closest to what you feel the majority of the researchers in your institution would make, acting in their role as researcher rather than as a "committee of one"? _____ (Please write in the number of the response.)

IF YOU WOULD LIKE TO MAKE ANY COMMENTS ON ANY PART OF QUESTION 46, please use the following space: _____
_____
_____
_____

ORGANIZATIONS WHICH AFFECT YOUR INSTITUTION

47. Sometimes organizations are able to influence the internal practices of other organizations.

    A. In column A below, place an X opposite all organizations that have influenced the effective policy of your institution with respect to the ethical aspects of clinical research.

    B. In column B below, place an X opposite the organization that has exerted the most influence on the effective policy of your institution with respect to the ethical aspects of clinical research.

List of Organizations	A Influenced Your Institution	B Most Influence On Your Institution
1. National Institutes of Health	( )	( )
2. Food and Drug Administration	( )	( )
3. National Science Foundation	( )	( )
4. Congressional Committees (Please specify)		
a. _____	( )	( )
b. _____	( )	( )
5. Other Federal Agencies (Please specify)		
a. _____	( )	( )
b. _____	( )	( )
6. American Medical Association	( )	( )
7. Voluntary organizations dedicated to the protection of human rights (e.g., ACLU; please specify)		
a. _____	( )	( )
b. _____	( )	( )
8. City or municipal government	( )	( )
9. County government	( )	( )
10. State government	( )	( )
11. Churches or religious organizations	( )	( )
12. Other institutions which do clinical research	( )	( )
13. Insurance companies	( )	( )
14. Other (please specify)		
a. _____	( )	( )
b. _____	( )	( )
15. None	( )	( )

48. Has any organization encouraged your institution to lessen the stringency of its controls over the ethical aspects of clinical research?

      ( ) a. Yes
      ( ) b. No

   48A. IF YES, please list the name(s) of any such organizations:

      1. _____
      2. _____

49. Has your institution actively sought advice on the ethical aspects of clinical research from representatives of any other organization(s)?

      ( ) a. Yes
      ( ) b. No

   49A. IF YES, please list the organization(s) from which your institution has sought advice:

      1. _____
      2. _____

50. Has your institution attempted to influence any other organization on the subject of the ethical aspects of clinical research?

      ( ) a. Yes
      ( ) b. No

   50A. IF YES, please list the organizations your institution has sought to influence:

      1. _____
      2. _____

51. Considering other organizations in the U.S. of the same general type as yours, please name the one(s) - up to three - which you judge to be doing, scientifically speaking, the highest quality clinical research:

Name of organization(s): 1. _____
                             2. _____
                             3. _____

52. What is your best estimate of the total sum, including grants from outside sources, budgeted by your institution for all activities in the current fiscal year?

                                                $_____

53. What is your best estimate of the sum, including grants from outside sources, budgeted by your institution in the current fiscal year for all research (that is, clinical and other)?

54. Approximately what proportion of the money reported in question 53 comes from the Public Health Service? (Check only one)

```
( ) a.  All or almost all
( ) b.  About three-fourths
( ) c.  About half
( ) d.  About one-fourth
( ) e.  None or almost none
```

55. What is the approximate number of people in your institution who do clinical research? Count only principal investigators and their main colleagues. _____ researchers

BACKGROUND INFORMATION

We would like to conclude this questionnaire with a few brief questions about yourself and your background.

56. Are you a member of the institutional review committee?

```
( ) a.  Yes
( ) b.  No
```

56A. IF YES TO QUESTION 56, please answer the following two questions:

56A.1. Do you hold any special position on the institutional review committee (such as chairman or executive secretary)?

```
( ) a.  Yes
( ) b.  No
```

IF YES TO 56A.1., please specify: _____

56A.2. How long have you been a member of the institutional review committee? (Please write in the number of years): _____ years

56B. IF NO TO QUESTION 56, do you have any other formal affiliation with the institutional review committee (i.e., grants administrator, observer, etc.)?

```
( ) 1.  Yes
( ) 2.  No
```

IF YES TO 56B, please specify: _____

57. In which of the following activities do you engage
(either in this institution or elsewhere)? (Check <u>all</u> that
apply)

      ( ) a. Laboratory research using only human materials,
            not directly using human subjects
      ( ) b. Research using human subjects
      ( ) c. Treatment of patients
      ( ) d. Other (please specify) _____

IF YOU CHECKED "a" or "b" IN QUESTION 57, please answer
the following six questions:

57A. Are you presently engaged in a clinical research
project?

      ( ) 1. Yes
      ( ) 2. No

57B. In what field or specialty do you do most of your
clinical research? _____ _____

57C. How many articles reporting your original clinical
research results have you published in the past <u>five</u> years
(not counting abstracts)? _____ articles

57D. Scientists are sometimes anticipated by others in
the presentation of research findings. That is, after
they have started work on a problem, another scientist
publishes its solution. With respect to all of your research, clinical and otherwise, how often has this happened to you in your career? (Please exclude cases where
a solution to your problem was published <u>before</u> you started your own work.)

      ( ) 1. Never
      ( ) 2. Once or twice
      ( ) 3. 3 to 5 times
      ( ) 4. More than 5 times

57E. How concerned are you that you might be anticipated
in your current clinical research?

      ( ) 1. Not presently engaged in clinical research
      ( ) 2. Very concerned
      ( ) 3. Moderately concerned
      ( ) 4. Slightly concerned
      ( ) 5. Not at all concerned

57F. Are there many of your colleagues who are concerned that they might be anticipated in their current clinical research?

( ) 1. I am aware of quite a few.
( ) 2. I am aware of some.
( ) 3. I am not aware of any.

58. Please give below your <u>official title(s)</u> in this institution and the <u>number of years you have held the title(s)</u> (if you have more than one, please list <u>up to three</u>):

a. _____ _____ years
b. _____ _____ years
c. _____ _____ years

58A. How long have you been a member of this institution? (Please write in the number of years): _____ years

59. What is your highest academic degree? _____

59A. From what institution did you receive your highest academic degree? _____

59B. <u>IF YOU ARE AN M.D.</u>, what is your specialty? _____
_____

59C. <u>IF YOUR HIGHEST DEGREE WAS PH.D., M.A., OR M.S.</u>, in what academic discipline did you earn the degree? _____
_____

60. What was your age at your last birthday? _____ years old

61. How would you characterize yourself politically at the present time?

( ) a. Left
( ) b. Liberal
( ) c. Middle of the road
( ) d. Moderately conservative
( ) e. Strongly conservative
( ) f. Other (please specify) _____
_____

62. In what religion were you raised and what is your present religious preference?

		Religion In Which Raised	Present Religious Preference
a.	Protestant (specify denomination) _____	( )	( )
b.	Roman Catholic	( )	( )
c.	Jewish (please specify) _____	( )	( )
d.	Other (please specify) _____		
e.	No religious affiliation	( )	( )

62A. Do you consider yourself:

( ) 1. Deeply religious
( ) 2. Moderately religious
( ) 3. Largely indifferent to religion
( ) 4. Basically opposed to religion

63. What is your current marital status?

( ) a. Single
( ) b. Married
( ) c. Separated
( ) d. Divorced
( ) e. Widowed

63A. Do you have any children?

( ) 1. Yes
( ) 2. No

64. Some of your colleagues in different institutions with whom we have talked about this questionnaire indicated a desire to discuss some or all of the questions with one or more of their local colleagues. We encouraged them to do so if they wished. It is important, however, for us to know whether the responses you have made here are your own or represent the product of a group effort. Please check <u>one</u> of the following:

( ) a. I did not consult with anyone on any questions in the questionnaire.

( ) b. I consulted with one or more others on factual questions about my institution (such as question 53) but did not consult on questions requesting a personal opinion (such as question 41).

( ) c. I consulted with one or more others on both factual questions about my institution and questions requesting a personal opinion.

( ) d. Other (please specify) _____

_____

_____

65. Since, as we noted in our cover letter, you may not be the person to whom this questionnaire was originally sent, we ask you to give us your name here. Again, let us emphasize that your replies will be held in strictest confidence. No one besides the immediate Columbia researchers will be able to identify your responses, and neither your identity nor that of your institution will be revealed. (<u>PLEASE PRINT</u>): _____

Thank you very much for your cooperation. Should you wish to add further comments, occasioned or provoked by this questionnaire, we shall appreciate them.

APPENDIX II
INTENSIVE TWO-INSTITUTION
INTERVIEW SCHEDULE

1. Are you presently or have you within the past year engaged in bio-medical research using human subjects <u>in this institution</u>?

    ( ) a. Presently engaged
    ( ) b. Within past year, but not now
    ( ) c. Have not been so engaged for over a year

    <u>IF PRESENTLY ENGAGED IN RESEARCH</u>, go to Question 2.

    <u>IF DID RESEARCH WITHIN THE PAST YEAR, BUT NOT NOW,</u> go on to Question 4.

    <u>IF NO RESEARCH FOR OVER A YEAR</u>, terminate the interview.

2. In how many research projects are you presently engaged in this institution? _____ projects

    2A. Since we are going to be referring to each of your research projects for a while, could you please give a brief name to each project for purposes of identification?

    1. _____
    2. _____
    3. _____
    4. _____
    5. _____
    6. _____
    7. _____
    8. _____

3. <u>FOR EACH RESEARCH PROJECT</u> in which you are presently engaged in this institution, please answer the following questions:

    3A. <u>For each project</u>: How many peers among your colleagues (including Ph.D.'s but not including interns), regardless of whether they are members of this institution or not, work with you on the research you do in this institution?

                              <u>Projects</u>

    1.____   2.____   3.____   4.____   5.____   6.____   7.____   8.____

3A.1. Can you give me the names of the colleagues
       working with you on each project?

<u>Projects</u>

1._____ 2._____

3._____ 4._____

5._____ 6._____

7._____ 8._____

3A.2. <u>For each project</u>: Will any of these colleagues
       you have named be joint authors with you on pa-
       pers resulting from your current research?

       ( ) a. Yes
       ( ) b. No

       <u>IF YES</u>, place an * next to the names for each
       project.

3A.3. <u>For each project</u>: Is any of those you have
named, including yourself, the leader of the
research group(s), or do you consider your
research group(s) to be a collaboration of
equals?

IF YES, place a √ next to the leader(s).
<u>IF COLLABORATION OF EQUALS</u>, circle the project
number.
<u>IF OTHER</u>, place an (x) next to the project
number.

3B. <u>For each project</u>: How many interns, medical students, or graduate students work with you?

<u>Projects</u>

1.____ 2.____ 3.____ 4.____ 5.____ 6.____ 7.____ 8.____

3B.1. <u>For each project</u>: Can you give me the names of
those interns, medical students or graduate
students?

<u>Projects</u>

1._____ 2._____

3._____ 4._____

5._____ 6._____

7._____ 8._____

3B.2. <u>For each project</u>: Will any of these interns,
<u>medical students</u> or graduate students be joint
authors with you on papers resulting from your
current research? (Place an * next to the
names.)

3C. For each project: During the past year, roughly how many times a month, on the average, have you gone to other researchers in your institution who are not collaborators with you on the project to discuss the project? (Those with whom you discuss the project in question may be collaborators on one or more of your other projects, although not on this project.)

Projects

1.____ 2.____ 3.____ 4.____ 5.____ 6.____ 7.____ 8.____

    3C.1. IF AT ALL FOR ANY PROJECT: For each project, with whom have you had such discussions?

Projects

1._____ 2._____

3._____ 4._____

5._____ 6._____

7._____ 8._____

3D. What three characteristics do you most want to know about another researcher before entering into a collaborative relationship with him?

    1. _____
    2. _____
    3. _____

3E. For each of the above projects in which human subjects are utilized: approximately what percentage
of the following categories of people are involved
as subjects?

Projects

1   2   3   4   5   6   7   8

___%___%___%___%___%___%___%___% a. Patients for whom it is
hoped the investigation
will have immediate therapeutic benefits

___%___%___%___%___%___%___%___% b. Patients for whom the investigation may have even-
tual therapeutic benefits,
but who are primarily subjects of scientific re-
search

___%___%___%___%___%___%___%___% c. Patients whose condition
is unrelated to the in-
vestigation

___%___%___%___%___%___%___%___% d. You, yourself, or other
researchers

___%___%___%___%___%___%___%___% e. Medical students
___%___%___%___%___%___%___%___% f. Para-medical personnel or
other employees of the in-
stitution (e.g., nurses,
laboratory personnel)

___%___%___%___%___%___%___%___% g. Prisoners
___%___%___%___%___%___%___%___% h. Normal volunteers (of any
type)

___%___%___%___%___%___%___%___% i. Other

3F. For each project in which patients are involved as
subjects, roughly what percentage of the subjects are:

Projects

1   2   3   4   5   6   7   8

___%___%___%___%___%___%___%___% a. Private patients
___%___%___%___%___%___%___%___% b. Semi-private patients
___%___%___%___%___%___%___%___% c. Ward patients
___%___%___%___%___%___%___%___% d. Clinic patients
___%___%___%___%___%___%___%___% e. Referred out-patients

___%___%___%___%___%___%___%___% a. Children under 13 years
of age
___%___%___%___%___%___%___%___% b. Persons aged 13-21
___%___%___%___%___%___%___%___% c. People beyond 65 years
of age
___%___%___%___%___%___%___%___% d. Terminal patients
___%___%___%___%___%___%___%___% e. Chronically ill patients

3G. <u>For each project in which patients are involved as</u>
<u>subjects,</u> are the patients who are involved as sub-
jects your patients, the patients of other physicians,
or what? (Check <u>all</u> that apply)

<u>1   2   3   4   5   6   7   8</u>

( ) ( ) ( ) ( ) ( ) ( ) ( ) ( )   a. Your patients
( ) ( ) ( ) ( ) ( ) ( ) ( ) ( )   b. Other physicians' pa-
                                        tients
( ) ( ) ( ) ( ) ( ) ( ) ( ) ( )   c. Ward or clinic patients
                                        of the house staff
( ) ( ) ( ) ( ) ( ) ( ) ( ) ( )   d. Other

    3G.1. IF OTHER PHYSICIANS' PATIENTS ARE USED: Can
          you give me the names of the physicians whose
          patients are involved in each of your studies?

<u>Projects</u>

1   2   3   4   5   6   7   8

____ ____ ____ ____ ____ ____ ____ ____
____ ____ ____ ____ ____ ____ ____ ____
____ ____ ____ ____ ____ ____ ____ ____
____ ____ ____ ____ ____ ____ ____ ____
____ ____ ____ ____ ____ ____ ____ ____
____ ____ ____ ____ ____ ____ ____ ____

<u>LET'S MOVE NOW TO THE AREA OF RISKS VS. BENEFITS:</u>

3H. For each project in which humans are involved as subjects: Assuming that "risk" is defined as danger to
the subject above and beyond that to which he is already exposed as a patient or as a normal, healthy
person, how much risk is involved for the subjects
who are at risk?

    <u>Projects</u>

<u>1   2   3   4   5   6   7   8</u>

( ) ( ) ( ) ( ) ( ) ( ) ( ) ( ) a. A large amount of risk for
                                      the subjects who are at risk
( ) ( ) ( ) ( ) ( ) ( ) ( ) ( ) b. A moderate amount of risk
                                      for the subjects who are at
                                      risk
( ) ( ) ( ) ( ) ( ) ( ) ( ) ( ) c. Some risk for the subjects
                                      who are at risk
( ) ( ) ( ) ( ) ( ) ( ) ( ) ( ) d. Very little risk for the
                                      subjects who are at risk
( ) ( ) ( ) ( ) ( ) ( ) ( ) ( ) e. No subjects are at risk

3I.   In your estimation, how significant for the advancement of medical knowledge is each of your projects?

(Check only one category for each project)

Projects

1   2   3   4   5   6   7   8

( ) ( ) ( ) ( ) ( ) ( ) ( ) ( ) a. If successful, it will be
an outstanding contribu-
tion.
( ) ( ) ( ) ( ) ( ) ( ) ( ) ( ) b. It will be a highly significant contribution.
( ) ( ) ( ) ( ) ( ) ( ) ( ) ( ) c. It will be a greater than
average contribution.
( ) ( ) ( ) ( ) ( ) ( ) ( ) ( ) d. It will be a modest, but
important, contribution.
( ) ( ) ( ) ( ) ( ) ( ) ( ) ( ) e. It will contribute something.
( ) ( ) ( ) ( ) ( ) ( ) ( ) ( ) f. Other

3I.1. In your estimation, what is the probability
that each project will be successful?

Projects

1   2   3   4   5   6   7   8

_____ _____ _____ _____ _____ _____ _____ _____

THIS BRINGS US NOW TO THE AREA OF POSSIBLE THERAPEUTIC BENE-
FITS, EITHER FOR THE SUBJECTS OF YOUR RESEARCH, FOR OTHERS,
OR FOR BOTH:

3J.   For each project in which humans are involved: If
successful, do you feel, for those subjects who are
at risk, that the research will provide any long or
short-term therapeutic benefits?

(Check only one category for each project)

Projects

1   2   3   4   5   6   7   8

( ) ( ) ( ) ( ) ( ) ( ) ( ) ( ) a. Yes, great therapeutic
benefit
( ) ( ) ( ) ( ) ( ) ( ) ( ) ( ) b. Yes, some benefit
( ) ( ) ( ) ( ) ( ) ( ) ( ) ( ) c. Yes, but only minor benefit
( ) ( ) ( ) ( ) ( ) ( ) ( ) ( ) d. Little or no benefit

3K. Once again, if the project is successful, how about therapeutic benefits for others?

(Check only one category for each project)

Projects

<u>1   2   3   4   5   6   7   8</u>

( ) ( ) ( ) ( ) ( ) ( ) ( ) ( ) a. Yes, great therapeutic benefit for others

( ) ( ) ( ) ( ) ( ) ( ) ( ) ( ) b. Yes, some benefit for others

( ) ( ) ( ) ( ) ( ) ( ) ( ) ( ) c. Yes, but only minor benefit for others

( ) ( ) ( ) ( ) ( ) ( ) ( ) ( ) d. Little or no benefit for others

4. Have you yourself ever been a subject in a bio-medical research study, not including practice procedures in medical school?

   ( ) a. Yes
   ( ) b. No

IF YES:

    4A. Did the study expose you to any risk?

   ( ) a. Yes
   ( ) b. No

    4B. Did you derive any therapeutic benefits?

   ( ) a. Yes
   ( ) b. No

5. Have you ever found yourself becoming involved emotionally with the people serving as subjects in your research to an extent greater than you deem desirable for a researcher?

   ( ) a. Yes
   ( ) b. No

IF YES: Under what circumstances? _____

_____

_____

_____

_____

6. <u>IF M.D.</u>: How many times in the past month have you gone to another physician in this institution to confer, formally or informally, on a therapeutic problem? _____ times

   6A. <u>IF AT ALL</u>: With whom did you confer?

   _____
   _____
   _____
   _____
   _____
   _____

7. <u>IF M.D.</u>: How many times in the past month has another physician in this institution come to you to confer, formally or informally, on one of his cases or therapeutic problems? _____ times

   7A. <u>IF AT ALL</u>: Who has come to you?

   _____
   _____
   _____
   _____
   _____
   _____

8. Sometimes conducting research on humans can confront an investigator with serious ethical dilemmas, the solutions to which are not always clear. During the past year, how many times have you discussed with one of your colleagues in this institution the ethical issues involved in the utilization of human subjects or an ethical dilemma present in your own research? _____ times

   8A. In general terms, not connected with your own research? _____ times

      8A.1. <u>IF AT ALL</u>: With whom have you discussed these issues?

      _____
      _____
      _____
      _____
      _____

   8B. As they have arisen in your own research? _____ times

      8B.1. <u>IF AT ALL</u>: With whom have you discussed these issues?

      _____
      _____
      _____
      _____
      _____

9. During the past year, how many times a month, on the average, have you had lunch with one or more of your colleagues (that is, researchers and/or physicians not doing research) from this institution? _____ times

    9A. IF AT ALL: With whom? _____
    _____
    _____
    _____
    _____
    _____

10. During the past year, how many times have you gotten together socially with one or more of your colleagues (that is, researchers and/or physicians not doing research) from this institution - visiting each other's homes, going to the theatre, parties, etc.? _____ times

    10A. IF AT ALL: With whom? _____
    _____
    _____
    _____
    _____

11. Would you please name the three physicians, whether in this institution or not, with whom you are most friendly?

    _____
    _____
    _____

SOME PROPOSED CLINICAL INVESTIGATIONS FOR REVIEW:

   The following are two hypothetical research proposals. Please assume that these proposed clinical investigations have never been conducted before - that is, they would not be replications of research already done (even if you know that either of them actually has been done before). With respect to each, we would like to know, in the hypothetical case that you constituted an institutional review "committee of one," what decision you would make after reviewing the proposals.

12. A researcher plans to study bone metabolism in children suffering from a serious bone disease. He intends to determine the degree of appropriation of calcium into the bone by using radioactive calcium. In order to make an adequate comparison, he intends to use some healthy children as controls, and he plans to obtain the consent of the parents of both groups of children after explaining to them the nature and purposes of the investigation and the short- and long-term risks to their children. Evidence from animals and earlier studies in humans indicates that the size of the radioactive dose to be administered here would only very slightly (say, by 5-10 chances in a million) increase the probability of the subjects involved contracting leukemia or experiencing other problems in the long run. While there is no definitive data as yet on the incidence of leukemia in children, a number of doctors and statistical sources indicate that the rate is about 250/million in persons under 18 years of age. Assume for the purposes of this question that the incidence of the bone disease being discussed is about the same as that for leukemia in children under 18 years of age. The investigation, if successful, would add greatly to medical knowledge regarding this particular bone disease, but the administration of radioactive calcium would not be of immediate therapeutic benefit for either group of children. The results of the investigation may, however, eventually benefit the group of children suffering from the bone disease. Please assume for the purposes of this question that there is no other method that would produce the data the researcher desires. The researcher is known to be highly competent in this area.

Hypothetically assuming that you constitute an institutional review "committee of one," and that the proposed investigation has never been done before, please check the lowest probability that you would consider acceptable for your approval of the proposed investigation. (Choose only one)

( ) 1. If the chances are 1 in 10 that the investigation will lead to an important medical discovery

(,) 2. If the chances are 3 in 10 that the investigation will lead to an important medical discovery

( ) 3. If the chances are 5 in 10 that the investigation will lead to an important medical discovery

( ) 4. If the chances are 7 in 10 that the investigation will lead to an important medical discovery

( ) 5. If the chances are 9 in 10 that the investigation will lead to an important medical discovery

( ) 6. Place a check here if you feel that, as the proposal stands, the researcher should not attempt the investigation, no matter what the probability that an important medical discovery will result.

COULD YOU PLEASE EXPLAIN YOUR ANSWER: _____
_____
_____
_____
_____

13. A researcher proposes to study pulmonary function in
adults under anesthesia for routine hernia repair. In order
to complete the necessary measurements for the investigation,
he would keep the patients under the anesthesia for an additional half hour. The completion of the investigation at
this particular time would result in an important increase
in medical knowledge of the effects of anesthesia on pulmonary function. As a result of additional time under anesthesia,
it is likely that the probability of post-operative complications such as atelectasis (collapse of some pulmonary tissue)
and pneumonia would increase slightly.

Hypothetically assuming that you constitute an institutional review "committee of one," and that the proposed research has never been done before, would you:

( ) 1. Approve the proposal as it stands?
( ) 2. Require some revisions in the proposal before
        you would approve it?
( ) 3. Reject the proposal?

13A. IF YOU CHECKED "2" ABOVE, what revisions or changes
would you require in the proposal before you would approve
it and why? _____
_____
_____
_____
_____
_____

13B. IF YOU CHECKED "3" ABOVE, why would you reject the
proposal? _____
_____
_____
_____
_____
_____

ON A SOMEWHAT DIFFERENT SUBJECT NOW:

14. How often during the past year has the question of ethics come to your attention under each of the following circumstances?

    14A. In connection with the practice of medicine?
                                      _____ times

        IF AT ALL: Can you give an example? _____
        _____
        _____

    14B. In connection with the use of human subjects in biomedical research? _____ times

        IF AT ALL: Can you give an example? _____
        _____

15. It is the policy of the Public Health Service that no grant, award, or contract for the support of research involving human subjects shall be made unless the research is given initial and continuing review and approval by an appropriate committee of the applicant institution. This review should insure that (a) the rights and welfare of the individuals involved are adequately protected, (b) the methods used to obtain informed consent are adequate and appropriate, and (c) the risks to the individual are outweighed by the potential benefits to him or by the importance of the knowledge to be gained.

    15A. Are you familiar with this policy?

        ( ) a. Yes
        ( ) b. No

    15B. Do you think that your research, if it involved human subjects, should be subject to the review and approval of your professional peers?

        ( ) a. Yes
        ( ) b. No

    COMMENTS: _____
                 _____

    15B.1. IF YES, do you think qualified laymen (such as lawyers) should also serve on review and approval committees?

        ( ) a. Yes
        ( ) b. No

    COMMENTS: _____
                 _____

16. The Public Health Service policy also states that: "An individual should generally be accepted as a research subject only after he, or his legally authorized guardian or next of kin, has consented to his participation in the research. Such consent is valid, however, only if the individual is first given a fair explanation of the procedures to be followed, their possible benefits and attendant hazards and discomforts, and the reasons for pursuing the research and its general objectives."

Do you feel that this part of the policy is:

( ) a. Intolerably restrictive?
( ) b. More restrictive than desirable?
( ) c. About right?
( ) d. Not strict enough?

COMMENTS: _____
_____

16A. How do you view the implementation of the PHS policy (as embodied in the two statements above) by the review committee in this institution?

( ) a. Intolerably restrictive
( ) b. More restrictive than desirable
( ) c. About right
( ) d. Not strict enough

COMMENTS: _____
_____

17. Do you have any comments on your own experiences with the review committee?

COMMENTS: _____
_____
_____
_____

UP TO THIS POINT OUR QUESTIONS HAVE BEEN QUITE STRUCTURED. NOW WE'RE GETTING INTO AN AREA ABOUT WHICH WE KNOW RELATIVELY LITTLE. THEREFORE, THE NEXT FEW QUESTIONS WE'LL BE ASKING WILL BE MORE OPEN-ENDED.

18. We have been discussing some of your attitudes toward research using human subjects. Can you remember when you first became aware of the issues involved in the use of human subjects in research? _____
_____
_____
_____
_____
_____

18A. Under what circumstances did you first become aware?

_____
_____
_____
_____

18B. Do you remember your reaction? _____

_____
_____
_____

19. Did you have any experiences before medical school which made you aware of the issues involved in the use of human subjects in research?

      ( ) a. Yes
      ( ) b. No

19A. IF YES, can you describe these experiences? _____

_____
_____
_____

20. In medical school, were there any courses or seminars especially devoted to the issues involved in the use of human subjects in research?

      ( ) a. Yes
      ( ) b. No

20A. IF YES, can you remember what issues were discussed?

_____
_____
_____

21. In medical school, did these issues come up when you and your peers were doing practice procedures on each other or doing various procedures on animals?

      ( ) a. Yes
      ( ) b. No

21A. IF YES, how or under what circumstances? _____

_____
_____
_____

22.   In medical school, did these issues ever arise during discussion of specific research projects which you read about or learned of in class?

        ( ) a. Yes
        ( ) b. No

  22A.   IF YES, how did the issues arise and what was discussed? _____

_____

_____

_____

23.   IF YOU HAVE BEEN A RESEARCH SUBJECT YOURSELF: Earlier in the interview you indicated that you had been a subject in a bio-medical research study. Was this during medical school?

        ( ) a. Yes
        ( ) b. No

  23A.   IF NO, when was it? _____

  23B.   Did your own experience as a research subject make you aware of the issues involved in the use of human subjects?

          ( ) a. Yes
          ( ) b. No

    23B.1.   IF YES, how? _____

_____

_____

_____

24.   In medical school, did you yourself conduct any studies involving human subjects or participate in any such projects as a co-researcher?

        ( ) a. Yes
        ( ) b. No

  24A.   IF YES, how were the issues we've been speaking about dealt with then? _____

_____

_____

_____

24B.   IF YES, was it in medical school that you first started being seriously active in research?

   ( ) a. Yes
   ( ) b. No

   24B.1. IF YES, in what year in medical school did you become seriously active? _____ year

   24B.2. IF NO, when did you start being seriously active in research? _____

   _____

   _____

25. Did you have any other experiences while in medical school which were important in forming your attitudes toward the use of humans in research?

   ( ) a. Yes
   ( ) b. No

   25A. IF YES, can you describe them briefly? _____

   _____

   _____

   _____

26. Did any of these issues with respect to human subjects come up in some new way in your clinical experience during your internship or residency years?

   ( ) a. Yes
   ( ) b. No

   26A. IF YES, how did these issues arise in a new way?

   _____

   _____

27. When you began doing your own research, were there any particular experiences which you feel changed or developed your attitudes concerning the ethical issues involved in the use of humans in research?

   ( ) a. Yes
   ( ) b. No

   27A. IF YES, what happened and how did you react? _____

   _____

   _____

   _____

28. Have you heard any lectures or talks or read any papers or books which especially helped you to develop your opinions in this area?

      ( ) a. Yes
      ( ) b. No

  28A. <u>IF YES</u>, can you tell us what it was that you found helpful? _____

_____

_____

_____

29. Now, out of all the things we've been discussing, what do you think had the greatest influence on the development of your attitudes toward the use of human subjects in research?

_____

_____

_____

<u>MOVING AGAIN TO A DIFFERENT TOPIC</u>:

30. How many articles reporting your original research results (including co-authored articles) have you published in the past <u>five</u> years? _____ papers

31. Have you ever won a prize, special award, or been elected to an honorary scientific society for your research accomplishments?

      ( ) a. Yes
      ( ) b. No

32. How easy do you find it to obtain grants to support the research you wish to do? (Check only <u>one</u>)

      ( ) a. I have <u>never</u> tried to obtain a research grant.
      ( ) b. I have <u>always</u> obtained support for the research I wish to do.
      ( ) c. I have <u>usually</u> obtained support.
      ( ) d. I have <u>seldom</u> obtained support.
      ( ) e. I have <u>never</u> obtained support.

33. In the last two decades, the amount of research produced has been increasing rapidly. As you see it, at what rate is your <u>primary</u> research specialty growing compared to the average rate of growth of other specialties in medicine? (Check only <u>one</u>)

 ( ) a. Much faster
 ( ) b. Somewhat faster
 ( ) c. At about the same rate
 ( ) d. Much more slowly or not at all

34. Scientists are sometimes anticipated by others in the presentation of research findings. That is, after they have started work on a problem, another scientist publishes its solution. With respect to all of your research, clinical or otherwise, how often has this happened to you in your career? (Please exclude cases where a solution to your problem was published <u>before</u> you started your own work.) (Check only <u>one</u>)

 ( ) a. Never
 ( ) b. Once or twice
 ( ) c. 3 to 5 times
 ( ) d. More than 5 times

 34A. <u>IF ANTICIPATED ONCE OR MORE</u>: In the most recent case, did you publish your results anyway? (Check <u>all</u> that apply)

  ( ) a. Yes, because my work is somewhat different from that previously published
  ( ) b. Yes, because publication of results of this type is desirable
  ( ) c. Yes, but for other reasons
  ( ) d. No

35. How concerned are you that you might be anticipated in your current research? (Check only <u>one</u>)

 ( ) a. Very concerned
 ( ) b. Moderately concerned
 ( ) c. Slightly concerned
 ( ) d. Not at all concerned

36. Would you feel quite safe in discussing your current research with other persons doing similar work in other institutions, or do you think it necessary to conceal the details of your work from some of them until you are ready to publish? (Check only <u>one</u>)

 ( ) a. I feel safe in discussing my work with <u>all</u> others.
 ( ) b. I feel safe in discussing my work with <u>most</u> others.
 ( ) c. I feel safe in discussing my work with only a few I can trust.

37. During an average year, what proportion of your total work time do you estimate that you spend on scientific research (as opposed to your practice, teaching, administration, etc.)? _____%

   37A. What proportion of your research is conducted at this institution? _____%

38. In addition to doing research, in which of the following activities do you engage in this institution or elsewhere? (Check all that apply)

        ( ) a. Treatment of patients
        ( ) b. Administration
        ( ) c. Teaching
        ( ) d. Other (please specify) _____

   38A. IF YOU TREAT PATIENTS, how do you feel your being a physician treating patients influences you when you do research using humans? (Check only one)

        ( ) a. It has the effect of assisting me in that research.
        ( ) b. It is supporting in some respects, hindering in others.
        ( ) c. It has the effect of hindering.
        ( ) d. It has no effect, direct or indirect.

        PLEASE EXPLAIN YOUR ANSWER VERY BRIEFLY: _____
        _____
        _____

   38B. IF YOU TREAT PATIENTS, how do you feel your being a researcher influences you when you treat patients? (Check only one)

        ( ) a. It has the effect of assisting me in the treatment of my patients.
        ( ) b. It is supporting in some respects, hindering in others.
        ( ) c. It has the effect of hindering.
        ( ) d. It has no effect, direct or indirect.

        PLEASE EXPLAIN YOUR ANSWER VERY BRIEFLY: _____
        _____
        _____

39. With which of the following statements do you most closely agree? (Check only one)

    ( ) a. This institution strongly encourages those who are qualified to engage in clinical research to do so.

    ( ) b. This institution moderately encourages those who are qualified to engage in clinical research to do so.

    ( ) c. This institution only slightly encourages those who are qualified to engage in clinical research to do so.

    ( ) d. This institution does not encourage those who are qualified to engage in clinical research to do so.

WE WOULD NOW LIKE TO CONCLUDE THIS INTERVIEW WITH A FEW BRIEF QUESTIONS ABOUT YOURSELF AND YOUR BACKGROUND:

40. Please give your official title(s) in this institution and the number of years you have held the title(s):

    a. _____ _____ years
    b. _____ _____ years
    c. _____ _____ years

    40A. Of what department are you a member? _____

    40B. How long have you been a member of this institution? _____ years

41. What is your highest academic degree? _____

    41A. In what year did you receive your highest degree? _____

    41B. From what institution did you receive your highest academic degree? _____

    41C. IF YOU ARE AN M.D., what is your specialty? _____

    41D. IF YOUR HIGHEST DEGREE WAS PH.D. OR OTHER, in what academic discipline did you earn the degree? _____

42. What college did you attend as an undergraduate? _____

43. What was your father's occupation at the time you entered college? _____

44. IF M.D. at the time you entered medical school, did you have any relatives (including members of your immediate family) who were doctors?

    ( ) a. Yes
    ( ) b. No

45. What was your age at your last birthday? _____ years old

46. Where were you born?   City _____
                           State _____
                           Country (if foreign) _____

47. Where was your father born?
                           City _____
                           State _____
                           Country (if foreign) _____

48. Where was your mother born?
                           City _____
                           State _____
                           Country (if foreign) _____

49. What is the predominant nationality of your ancestors?
_____

50. How would you characterize yourself politically at the present time?

      ( ) a. Left
      ( ) b. Liberal
      ( ) c. Middle of the road
      ( ) d. Moderately conservative
      ( ) e. Strongly conservative
      ( ) f. Other (please specify) _____
      _____

51. In what religion were you raised and what is your present religious preference?

		Religion In Which Raised	Present Religious Preference
a.	Protestant (specify denomination) _____	( )	( )
b.	Roman Catholic	( )	( )
c.	Jewish (please specify) _____	( )	( )
d.	Other (please specify) _____	( )	( )
e.	No religious affiliation	( )	( )

51A. Do you consider yourself:

        ( ) a. Deeply religious
        ( ) b. Moderately religious
        ( ) c. Largely indifferent to religion
        ( ) d. Basically opposed to religion

52. What is your current marital status?

        ( ) a. Single
        ( ) b. Married
        ( ) c. Separated
        ( ) d. Divorced
        ( ) e. Widowed

52A. Do you have any children?

        ( ) 1. Yes
        ( ) 2. No

53. Since we have also interviewed others in this institution and previously sent a questionnaire to your institution on this topic, we are interested in knowing whether you have discussed or have heard of any of our questions before this interview?

        ( ) a. Yes.
        ( ) b. No

    COMMENTS: _____

                  _____

54. Sex (interviewer checks)

        ( ) a. Male
        ( ) b. Female

55. Race (interviewer checks)

        ( ) a. White
        ( ) b. Negro
        ( ) c. Other (please specify) _____

INDEX